The Complete Keto
VEGETARIAN COOKBOOK

100 delicious and easy to make recipes with the nutritional value of every ingredient for simpler diet planning

7 days meal plan and shopping list

Sara Julian

INTRODUCTION

Congratulations on taking the first step towards a healthier lifestyle! This book was designed to give you a kickstart in your journey towards a keto vegetarian diet. For many people, making the transition can seem overwhelming. We're here to assure you: it's not as hard as it appears.

Our mission is to make this process as easy and as simple for you. To start off, we have designed a 7-day meal plan which explores the possibilities of what you can eat with a keto vegetarian diet. We have also provided a convenient grocery list for this 7-day meal plan.

The meal plan is just a preview of a full-on keto vegetarian diet, the objective of which is to assure you that you can still enjoy tasty and satisfying meals. Once you're ready to take the plunge, you can just pick any meal from the other recipes we have lovingly prepared for you. The recipes range from simple smoothies and salads that you can prepare in just a few minutes, to more involved recipes designed to expand your horizons in terms of cooking according to the diet.

Are you excited? Because we are. We're excited about how you're going to feel after the 7-day diet and for you to discover the benefits of a keto vegetarian diet. Always keep in mind that you're not depriving yourself. Instead, you're making the choice to eat meals that are better for your body. Making the shift to a keto vegetarian diet is a lifestyle choice, and we'll be glad to accompany you in your journey.

SARA JULIAN

INTRODUCTION 2

WHAT IS A KETOGENIC DIET?..6

WHAT DOES A KETOGENIC DIET DO TO OUR BODY?......................6

HOW CAN WE REACH KETOSIS?...7

WHAT ARE THE BENEFITS OF A KETOGENIC DIET? 8

HOW DO YOU MAKE THE SHIFT TO A KETOGENIC DIET SAFELY?.................9

WHAT IS A KETOGENIC VEGETARIAN DIET? 10

WHAT FOOD CAN BE EATEN IN A KETOGENIC VEGETARIAN DIET?.............11

7-DAY KETO VEGETARIAN MEAL PLAN...12

    SHOPPING LIST..12

DAY 1...14

    QUICHE 14

    RICOTTA AND WALNUT ZOODLES 15

    THICK AND CREAMY CURRY SOUP 16

DAY 2...18

    HIGH-PROTEIN OVERNIGHT OATS 18

    CAULIFLOWER SALAD WITH FETA CHEESE 19

    TOFU AND GREENS SOUP 20

DAY 3...21

    MUSHROOM AND ZUCCHINI FRITTATA 21

    ASPARAGUS AND TOFU STIR FRY 23

    ROASTED CAULIFLOWER SOUP 24

DAY 4...25

    YOGURT BOWL WITH NUTS AND SEEDS 25

    HIGH-PROTEIN CAULIFLOWER FLATBREAD 26

    BROCCOLI AND MUSHROOM IN CHEESE SAUCE 28

DAY 5...29

    OVERNIGHT COCONUT CHIA PUDDING...29

    CHEESY CREAM OF MUSHROOM SOUP 30

    ZUCCHINI AND CABBAGE SALAD 31

DAY 6...33

    SPINACH MUSHROOM FRITTATA 33

    KETO SUMMER SALAD 34

ASIAN EGG DROP SOUP 35

DAY 7 36

CURRIED TOFU SCRAMBLE WITH MUSHROOMS 37

GREEK-STYLE KETO SALAD 38

SPICY CAULIFLOWER SOUP 39

OTHER KETO VEGETARIAN RECIPES 41

EASY KETO BAGELS 42

ARUGULA SALAD WITH AVOCADO 43

KETO HASH BROWNS 44

ZOODLES IN PESTO SAUCE 45

ZOODLES IN ALFREDO SAUCE 47

ROASTED TOFU IN TAHINI 48

MIXED GREENS AND COCONUT SMOOTHIE 49

BAKED EGGS IN AVOCADO BOATS 50

CAULIFLOWER GRILLED CHEESE SANDWICH 51

TRIPLE GREEN SALAD WITH ASIAN DRESSING 52

KETO FALAFEL WITH TAHINI SAUCE 53

TOFU IN CREAM OF ASPARAGUS SOUP 55

EGG SALAD 56

KETO MUSHROOM PIZZA 57

HIGH-PROTEIN SPINACH SMOOTHIE 58

CREAM OF CAULIFLOWER SOUP 59

CREAM CHEESE SCRAMBLED EGGS 60

MEDITERRANEAN ZOODLES 61

ROASTED TOFU AND ASPARAGUS 62

KETO FRIED MAC AND CHEESE 63

PESTO MUG CAKE 64

CHEESY CAULIFLOWER GRITS 65

SESAME AND ALMOND ASIAN ZOODLES 67

VEGETABLE AND TOFU CURRY 68

CHEESY KETO WAFFLES 69

SPICY ROASTED TOFU IN SOFT TACOS 71

HIGH-PROTEIN GRANOLA BARK 72

BASIC MUSHROOM OMELET 73

FRIED ZUCCHINI PATTIES WITH PESTO SAUCE 75

STUFFED PORTOBELLO PIZZAS 76

CHEESY ROASTED BROCCOLI AND CAULIFLOWER 77

TWO-CHEESE ASPARAGUS FRITTATA 78

ZOODLES PAD THAI 79

CHEESY BRUSSELS SPROUTS 81

QUICK CAPRESE SALAD 82

CHEESY CAULIFLOWER MASH 83

Simple Roasted Broccoli and Tofu 84
High-Protein Coconut and Chocolate Smoothie 85
Keto Vegetarian Lasagna 86
Keto-Friendly Pumpkin Soup 87
Teriyaki Tofu 88
Ricotta and Cheddar Cheese Fritters 90
Spinach and Ricotta Bake 91
Keto-Friendly Overnight Oats 92
Ricotta Dumplings in Tomato Sauce 93
Roasted Vegetables in Pesto 94
Keto Vegetarian Club Salad 95
Asparagus and Tofu Mash 96
Broccoli Cheese Fritters 97
Creamy Broccoli and Leek Soup 99
Baked Eggs in Collard Greens and Tomatoes 100
Creamy and Cheesy Cauliflower Rice 101
Spinach-Stuffed Portobello Mushrooms 102
Mexican-Style Cauliflower Rice 103
Arugula and Feta Cheese Salad 105
Ricotta-Stuffed Bell Peppers 106
Refreshing Green Smoothie 107
Keto Muffin Sandwich 108
Pumpkin and Ricotta Cheese Pancakes 109
Caprese-Style Omelet 110
Zucchini and Walnut Salad 111
Quick and Easy Keto Yogurt Bowl 112
Baked Ricotta Tarts 113
Hearty Vegetable Soup 115
Creamy Pumpkin Soup 116
Roasted Vegetables Smothered in Pesto and Ricotta 117
Keto-Friendly Three-Cheese Pizza 119
Eggplant Fritters in Tomato Sauce 120
Keto-Friendly Spinach Quiche 121
Five-Minute Broccoli Cheese Soup 122
Traditional-Style Mediterranean Salad 123
Cucumber and Dill Salad 124
Roasted Herbed Tofu and Mushrooms 125
Keto Waffles 126
Crispy Cauliflower Bites with Cream Cheese Dip 127
Cheesy Keto Bagels 129
Cream of Zucchini Soup 130
Creamy Two-Mushroom Soup 131
Spinach Feta Quiche 132

What is a ketogenic diet?

A ketogenic diet is easily described by two terms: low carbohydrates, and high fat. There is another characteristic of the diet – sufficient protein – that many sources forget to mention. In any case, the goal of the ketogenic diet is to replace the carbohydrates normally consumed in a traditional diet with equivalent calories from fats.

The ketogenic diet was first practices in the 1920s as a way to control epileptic seizures instead of taking medicine. As drugs became more effective, the diet became less popular until recent years. Scientific and mainstream interest in the diet was revived in the late 1990s because of a heavily publicized case of the use of the diet to treat epileptic seizures when traditional therapies have failed.

Nowadays, most people who practice the ketogenic diet do so to reap the other health benefits aside from epilepsy treatment. It has become one of the most popular diets and has enjoyed enduring popularity that has now spanned almost two decades.

What does a ketogenic diet do to our body?

On a traditional diet rich with carbohydrates, the body breaks down the complex carbohydrates into simple sugars. These simple sugars, colloquially known as glucose, play an important role in providing energy and fueling brain activity.

When there is little carbohydrates available to the body for energy production, it shifts into a mechanism in which the liver convers fat into fatty acids and ketones. These ketones practically take on the role glucose, fueling brain activity and providing energy for other bodily functions.

When your body enters this state -called 'ketosis' – it burns the body's fat stores much faster. This rapid fat consumption, along with the lowered insulin levels as a result of a low carbohydrate diet, result in the numerous health benefits that have made the ketogenic diet so popular.

How can we reach ketosis?

Ketosis is the state in which the body no longer has enough glycogen stored to break down into glucose and to fuel bodily functions. Because of this shortage, the body turns to another source of energy, which is fat. Reaching the state of ketosis results in faster fat burning, consequently making it easier to lose weight.

The fastest way to reach ketosis is to fast. By not consuming any food, the body consumes more and more of its energy storage in the form of both glycogen and fat. However, fasting may not be for everyone. For many people, switching to a ketogenic diet is a more sustainable option. By reducing carbohydrates and making the switch to a more fat-rich diet, the body can enter ketosis without running into a shortage of energy.

A way to reach ketosis faster is to increase your body's metabolism. This is typically done by performing moderate to heavy exercise. By consuming more energy, you can force your body to burn through its glycogen storage and start consuming fat. Paired with a ketogenic diet, regular exercise can quickly consumer your body's glycogen storage, which will not be replenished if you are on a low-carbohydrate diet.

What are the benefits of a ketogenic diet?

1. **Weight loss**

   If your primary objective for starting a keto diet is weight loss, then this is one of the easiest objectives to attain. Since ketosis speeds up the rate at which the body burns through the fat, all the fat stored in your body will be consumed much faster than if you were eating a carbohydrate-rich diet. Many people have reported a significant weight loss within the first two weeks of starting a ketogenic diet.

2. **Treats epilepsy**

   The primary reason for why the ketogenic diet was developed, treatment of epileptic seizures is still considered one of the best benefits of adopting a keto diet. This has been a well-documented phenomenon over several decades and has been supported by numerous medical tests. The ketogenic diet has even been shown to treat the seizures of patients who have already been non-responsive to drugs and other therapy methods.

3. Manages Type 2 Diabetes

   The mere fact that a ketogenic diet can help you shed excess fat already addresses one of the top indicators of Type 2 diabetes. The diet also requires that you manage your carbohydrate intake, which is recommended for people already suffering from diabetes or prediabetes. In a study published by NCBI, it was shown that 95% of diabetics who made the shift to a ketogenic diet were able to stop or reduce diabetes medication.

4. May also treat other diseases

   Based on some studies, the ketogenic diet has shown some efficacy in reducing the chances of developing heart disease, cancers, Alzheimer's disease, Parkinson's disease, and acne. While these cases aren't as well-documented, there is no denying that a ketogenic diet addresses many of the risk factors of these conditions such as obesity and high sugar intake.

How do you make the shift to a ketogenic diet safely?

Shifting to a ketogenic diet can be a pretty big lifestyle change for you. It's important to be aware that a ketogenic diet has its risks. You can be missing out on some essential nutrients that your body may need if you have a medical condition. It's also possible to end up with too much ketones in your blood – a condition called ketoacidosis, which is considered a medical emergency. Here are a few of our tips so you can safely make the shift.

1. Consult a medical professional

   There is no better way to understand the potential effects of adopting a ketogenic diet than for you to consult a medical service provider or a registered dietitian. While the keto diet is safe for most people, you may have an existing condition which may make your situation unique.

2. Be ready for the keto flu

   The first few days of the ketogenic diet are the hardest. Aside from the challenge of eating a completely different diet, you may also experience flu-like symptoms such as dizziness, stomach pains, nausea, cramps, and irritability. This is mostly the effect of mild dehydration, as your body's water retention is greatly reduced because of a lack of carbohydrates. This may also be the result of a lower level of sodium, potassium, and magnesium.

To remedy the effects of the keto flu, you must remember to always stay dehydrated. You can also consider taking supplements to make up for the lack of minerals. Sleep and exercise are equally important, so make sure you're still getting a healthy amount of both.

3. Listen to your body

    The great thing about the human body is that it lets you know if there's something wrong. In this regard, it is important to always keep listening to your body when you start on the keto diet. You may feel your energy levels lowering or your mental clarity suffering after a while. What's important is that you respond to these symptoms: eat a filling snack, take a break, or drink some water.

    Lastly, the keto diet isn't the only way to live a healthy lifestyle. If you find that eating a ketogenic diet is making you miserable, then you need to consider the possibility that it may not be for you. There is no shame in accepting this fact. It's more important that you don't develop a negative relationship with food and with your own body.

What is a ketogenic vegetarian diet?

A ketogenic vegetarian diet does away with meat derived from animals, on top of already eliminating high-carbohydrate source. There are several types of vegetarian diets, and you may a choice based on ethical, environmental, or medical considerations.

1. Lacto-ovo-vegetarians do not eat red meat, white meat, fish, or fowl but consume eggs and dairy products.

2. Ovo-vegetarians do not eat meat from animals and dairy products but eat eggs and egg products.
3. Lacto-vegetarians do not eat meat from animals as well as eggs and egg products. However, they consume dairy products.
4. Vegans do no eat meat or any other products derived from animals. This includes honey, gelatin, and any other animal byproducts. Vegans may also forego products that use leather, wool, or silk.

We have made an effort to cater to all these types of vegetarian diets in this cookbook. No matter what diet you have, you're bound to find recipes in this cookbook that appeal to you.

What food can be eaten in a ketogenic vegetarian diet?

1. Natural fats – Butter, olive oil, coconut oil, avocado oil
2. Eggs
3. Cheese – While most cheeses are vegetarian, there are some such as Parmesan, Gorgonzola, and Gruyere that use animal rennet during the production process. Double check if the cheese you are using is really vegetarian.
4. Vegetables that grow above the ground – Leafy vegetables such as spinach and kale, broccoli, cauliflower, zucchini, squash
5. Herbs and spices – Parsley, basil, oregano, paprika, cumin, ginger, garlic, chives
6. Nuts and seeds – Nuts and nut-derived products such as peanut butter and almond butter, almond flour, peanut flour, sunflower seeds, hemp seeds, poppy seeds
7. Coconut products – Coconut milk, coconut oil, desiccated coconut, coconut flour

7-DAY KETO VEGETARIAN MEAL PLAN

SHOPPING LIST

Item	Quantity
FRUITS AND VEGETABLES	
Avocado	1 piece
Asparagus	5 spears
Bell peppers	2 pieces
Broccoli	5 cups, chopped
Cabbage	1 head
Cauliflower	5 cups, chopped
Chili peppers	2 pieces
Coconut milk	4 cups; 1-liter pack
Cucumber	1 piece
Desiccated Coconut	2 tbsp
Garlic	2 bulbs
Ginger	1 piece
Green onion	1 piece
Green peppers	1 piece
Lemons	2 pieces
Lettuce	8 cups, chopped
Mustard greens	1 cup, chopped
Olives	3 pieces
Onion leeks	0.25 cup, chopped
Red onion	2 pieces
Spinach	4 cups
White mushroom	6 tbsp, sliced
White onion	4 pieces
Zucchini	3 pieces
Vegetable broth	3.5 cups
EGGS AND DAIRY PRODUCTS	
Cheddar	2 cups, shredded
Cream cheese	1 bar
Eggs	9 pieces
Feta cheese	2 cups

Greek yogurt	2 cups
Heavy cream	3 cups
Milk	1 cup
Mozzarella	1 cup
Protein powder	5 scoops
Ricotta	1/2 cup
FATS, OILS, AND VINEGARS	
Butter	12 tbsp; 2 bars
Balsamic vinegar	1 tbsp
Cider vinegar	1 tbsp
Coconut oil	4.5 tbsp
Olive oil	14 tbsp; 250mL bottle
Red wine vinegar	1 tbsp
Sesame oil	5 tbsp
SOY-BASED PRODUCTS	
Firm tofu	3 cups, cubes
Soft tofu	3 cups, cubes
Soy sauce	1 tbsp
SEEDS AND NUTS	
Almonds	0.5 tbsp
Chia seeds	0.5 tbsp
Peanuts	0.5 tbsp
Pecans	1.5 tbsp
Sesame seeds	1.5 tbsp
Sunflower seeds	1.5 tbsp
Walnuts	1 tbsp
HERBS, SPICES, AND SEASONING	
Basil	1 tbsp
Cilantro	1 tbsp
Cumin	0.5 tbsp
Curry powder	1.5 tbsp
Fish sauce	1.5 tbsp
Oregano	0.5 tbsp
Paprika	0.5 tbsp
Parsley	0.5 tbsp
Vanilla extract	0.5 tbsp

DAY 1

BREAKFAST	Spinach Quiche	512 cal
LUNCH	Ricotta and Walnut Zoodles	798 cal
DINNER	Thick and Creamy Curry Soup	631 cal

Quiche

INGREDIENTS	Protein	Fat	Carbs
1 cup spinach	0.86 g	0.12 g	1.09 g
2 eggs	11.05 g	8.37 g	0.63 g
1/2 cup cheddar, shredded	13.58 g	19.11 g	0.75 g
1 tbsp white onion, chopped	0.11 g	0.01 g	0.93 g
1 tbsp butter, melted	0.12 g	11.52 g	0.01 g
1/4 cup whole milk	1.92 g	1.99 g	2.92 g
1/2 tbsp garlic, chopped	0.27 g	0.02 g	1.42 g

Nutrition Facts

Amount per 264 g
1 serving (9.3 oz)

Calories 512
From fat 368

HappyForks.com

Amount	% Daily Value*	Amount	% Daily Value*
Total Fat 41.1g	63%	Total Carbohydrates 8g	3%
Saturated 22.2g	111%	Dietary Fiber 1g	4%
Trans Fat 1.2g		Sugars 4g	
Cholesterol 422mg	141%	Protein 28g	56%
Sodium 631mg	26%		
Calcium 54% • Iron 14%		Vitamin A 86% • Vitamin C 18%	

* Percent Daily Values are based on 2000 calorie diet. Your Daily Values may be higher or lower depending on your calorie needs.

1. Preheat the oven to 350 F.
2. In a medium-sized bowl, combine the eggs, spinach, shredded cheddar, white onion, garlic and milk. Whisk together until thoroughly mixed.
3. Brush the bottom and sides of a muffin pan with the melted butter.
4. Pour the egg mixture into the muffin pan.
5. Bake in the oven for about 30 minutes, or until the eggs have set at the top surface.
6. Remove the pan from the oven and allow to cool for 10 minutes before serving.

Ricotta and Walnut Zoodles

INGREDIENTS	Protein	Fat	Carbs
1 medium-sized zucchini	2.37 g	0.63 g	6.1 g
1/2 cup walnuts, ground	6.09 g	26.08 g	5.48 g
2 tbsp olive oil	0 g	27 g	0 g
1 tbsp lemon juice	0.05 g	0.04 g	1.06 g
1 tsp garlic, chopped	0.18 g	0.01 g	0.93 g
1/4 cup cheddar, shredded	7.93 g	11.16 g	0.44 g
1/4 cup ricotta cheese	6.98 g	8.05 g	1.88 g
1/4 cup Greek yogurt	2.55 g	0.1 g	0.9 g

Nutrition Facts

Amount per 401 g

1 serving (14.1 oz)

Calories 798

From fat 635

HappyForks.com

Amount	% Daily Value*	Amount	% Daily Value*
Total Fat 73.1g	112%	Total Carbohydrates 17g	6%
Saturated 17.9g	90%	Dietary Fiber 5g	19%
Trans Fat 0.4g		Sugars 7g	
Cholesterol 67mg	22%	Protein 26g	52%
Sodium 291mg	12%		
Calcium 46% • Iron 13%		Vitamin A 20% • Vitamin C 71%	

* Percent Daily Values are based on 2000 calorie diet. Your Daily Values may be higher or lower depending on your calorie needs.

INSTRUCTIONS:

1. Using a spiralizer or mandolin slicer, cut the zucchini into noodles or very thin strips.
2. In a large bowl, combine the sliced zucchini, cheddar, ricotta cheese, ground walnuts, and Greek yogurt.
3. In a separate, smaller bowl, combine the olive oil, lemon juice, and chopped garlic. Add a pinch of salt and pepper and whisk together.
4. Add the dressing to the salad right before serving. Toss thoroughly and serve right away.

Thick and Creamy Curry Soup

INGREDIENTS	Protein	Fat	Carbs
1/4 cup coconut milk	1.14 g	12.05 g	1.59 g
2 tbsp coconut oil	0 g	27.2 g	0 g
1/2 tbsp fish sauce	0.46 g	0 g	0.33 g
1/2 cup cauliflower, chopped	1.03 g	0.15 g	2.66 g
3/4 cup soft tofu, cubed	16.24 g	9.15 g	4.46 g
1 tbsp butter	0.12 g	11.52 g	0.01 g
1/4 tbsp ginger	0.03 g	0.01 g	0.27 g

1/2 tbsp curry powder	0.46 g	0.45 g	1.79 g
1/4 tbsp garlic, chopped	0.13 g	0.01 g	0.69 g
1/2 tbsp green peppers, chopped	0.04 g	0.01 g	0.22 g
1/4 tbsp cilantro, chopped	0.01 g	0 g	0.01 g

Nutrition Facts

Amount per 420 g
1 serving (14.8 oz)

Calories 631
From fat 518

HappyForks.com

	Amount	% Daily Value*	Amount	% Daily Value*
Total Fat 60.6g		93%	**Total Carbohydrates** 12g	4%
Saturated 43g		215%	Dietary Fiber 3g	14%
Trans Fat 0.5g			Sugars 3g	
Cholesterol 31mg		10%	**Protein** 20g	39%
Sodium 844mg		35%		
Calcium 33% • **Iron** 31%			**Vitamin A** 8% • **Vitamin C** 53%	

* Percent Daily Values are based on 2000 calorie diet. Your Daily Values may be higher or lower depending on your calorie needs.

INSTRUCTIONS:

1. In a saucepan, pre-heat the coconut oil over high heat. Add the ginger, garlic, and curry paste and cook for 1 to 2 minutes until fragrant.
2. Add the coconut milk and 1/4 cup of water. Allow to boil and simmer for 15 minutes.
3. Add the fish sauce, bell peppers, and tofu. Continue simmering for an additional 5 minutes while stirring.
4. Add the chopped cauliflower and cilantro. Simmer for an additional 5 minutes.
5. Turn off the heat. Add the butter and allow to melt into the curry before serving.

DAY 2

BREAKFAST	High-Protein Overnight Oats	734 cal
LUNCH	Cauliflower Salad with Feta Cheese	581 cal
DINNER	Tofu and Greens Soup	609 cal

High-Protein Overnight Oats

INGREDIENTS	Protein	Fat	Carbs
1 tbsp almonds, slivered	2.54 g	5.99 g	2.59 g
1/2 cup coconut milk	2.28 g	24.1 g	3.18 g
1 tbsp desiccated coconut	0.64 g	8.29 g	2.58 g
2 tbsp protein powder	10.06 g	3.77 g	4.07 g
1 tsp sunflower seeds	0.6 g	1.49 g	0.58 g
2 tbsp coconut oil	0 g	27.2 g	0 g
1/4 tbsp chia seeds	0.5 g	0.92 g	1.26 g
1/4 tsp vanilla extract	0 g	0 g	0.14 g

Nutrition Facts

Amount per 193 g
1 serving (6.8 oz)

Calories 734
From fat 610

HappyForks.com

	Amount	% Daily Value*	Amount	% Daily Value*
Total Fat	71.8g	110%	Total Carbohydrates 14g	5%
Saturated	53.3g	266%	Dietary Fiber 4g	17%
Trans Fat	0.1g		Sugars 2g	
Cholesterol	5mg	2%	Protein 17g	33%
Sodium	92mg	4%		
Calcium 19% • Iron 38%			Vitamin A 11% • Vitamin C 13%	

* Percent Daily Values are based on 2000 calorie diet. Your Daily Values may be higher or lower depending on your calorie needs.

INSTRUCTIONS:

1. Combine the protein powder, coconut oil, coconut milk, and vanilla extract in a blender. Blend until smooth.
2. Transfer the contents into an airtight container. To the same container, add the desiccated coconut, sunflower

seeds, and chia seeds. Mix thoroughly, cover, and leave overnight.

3. The following day, add the slivered almonds and serve

Cauliflower Salad with Feta Cheese

INGREDIENTS	Protein	Fat	Carbs
1/2 cup cauliflower, chopped	1.54 g	0.22 g	3.99 g
1/2 tbsp red onion, chopped	0.06 g	0.01 g	0.47 g
3 cup iceberg lettuce, shredded	1.94 g	0.3 g	6.42 g
1 tbsp red wine vinegar	0.01 g	0 g	0.04 g
2 1/2 tbsp olive oil	0 g	33.8 g	0 g
1/2 cup feta cheese, crumbled	10.66 g	15.96 g	3.07 g
1/2 cup Greek yogurt	5.1 g	0.2 g	1.8 g

Nutrition Facts

Amount per 475 g
1 serving (16.8 oz)

Calories 581
From fat 445

HappyForks.com

	Amount	% Daily Value*	Amount	% Daily Value*
Total Fat	50.5g	78%	Total Carbohydrates 16g	5%
Saturated	16.1g	80%	Dietary Fiber 4g	17%
Trans Fat	0g		Sugars 11g	
Cholesterol	69mg	23%	Protein 19g	39%
Sodium	754mg	31%		
Calcium	48% • Iron	11%	Vitamin A 28% • Vitamin C	75%

* Percent Daily Values are based on 2000 calorie diet. Your Daily Values may be higher or lower depending on your calorie needs.

INSTRUCTIONS:

1. Boil a pot of salted water and blanch the cauliflower for exactly 1 minute. Submerge immediately in ice water and strain on a colander.
2. In a large bowl, combine the cauliflower, iceberg lettuce, and red onion.

3. In a smaller bowl, whisk together the red wine vinegar, olive oil, and Greek yogurt. Add a pinch of salt and pepper.
4. Drizzle the dressing over the salad. Sprinkle with crumbled feta cheese.

Tofu and Greens Soup

INGREDIENTS	Protein	Fat	Carbs
1 cup spinach	0.86 g	0.12 g	1.09 g
1/2 cup mustard greens, chopped	0.8 g	0.12 g	1.31 g
1/2 cup coconut milk	2.28 g	24.1 g	3.18 g
1/2 cup vegetable broth	0 g	0 g	1.5 g
3 tbsp olive oil	0 g	27 g	0 g
1/2 tbsp white onion, chopped	0.06 g	0.01 g	0.47 g
1/4 tbsp ginger	0.03 g	0.01 g	0.27 g
1/4 tbsp garlic, chopped	0.13 g	0.01 g	0.69 g
1/2 tsp paprika	0.17 g	0.15 g	0.65 g
1/2 tsp cumin	0.2 g	0.24 g	0.49 g
3/4 cup soft tofu, cubed	12.18 g	6.86 g	3.35 g

Nutrition Facts

Amount per 512 g
1 serving (18.1 oz)

Calories 609
From fat 503

	Amount	% Daily Value*	Amount	% Daily Value*
	Total Fat 58.6g	90%	Total Carbohydrates 13g	4%
	Saturated 26.2g	131%	Dietary Fiber 3g	10%
	Trans Fat 0g		Sugars 3g	
	Cholesterol 0mg	0%	Protein 17g	33%
	Sodium 533mg	22%		
	Calcium 31% • Iron 46%		Vitamin A 91% • Vitamin C 51%	

* Percent Daily Values are based on 2000 calorie diet. Your Daily Values may be higher or lower depending on your calorie needs.

<u>**INSTRUCTIONS:**</u>

1. Pre-heat the olive oil in a medium-sized pot over high heat.
2. Add the paprika, cumin, and coriander and toast for about a minute.
3. Add the white onion, garlic, and ginger and sauté for 1 to 2 minutes.
4. Add the coconut milk and vegetable broth. Allow to boil and simmer for 10 minutes.
5. Add the spinach and mustard greens. Continue simmering until the greens have wilted.
6. Transfer the contents of the pot into a food processor or blender. Pulse until smooth.
7. Transfer the contents of the blender back into the pot and bring to a boil.
8. Add the cubed soft tofu and simmer for an additional10 minutes.
9. Serve while hot.

DAY 3

BREAKFAST	Mushroom and Zucchini Frittata	590 cal
LUNCH	Asparagus and Tofu Stir Fry	663 cal
DINNER	Roasted Cauliflower Soup	785 cal

Mushroom and Zucchini Frittata

INGREDIENTS	Protein	Fat	Carbs
1/2 medium zucchini, sliced	1.19 g	0.31 g	3.05 g
2 eggs	11.05 g	8.37 g	0.63 g
2 tbsp butter	0.24 g	23.04 g	0.02 g

1/2 cup white mushrooms, sliced	1.08 g	0.12 g	1.14 g
1/4 cup cheddar, shredded	6.8 g	9.57 g	0.38 g
1/2 tbsp garlic	0.27 g	0.02 g	1.42 g
1/2 tbsp white onion	0.06 g	0.01 g	0.47 g
1/2 cup bell peppers, sliced	0.4 g	0.08 g	2.13 g
1/4 cup heavy cream	0.62 g	11.1 g	0.84 g

Nutrition Facts

Amount per 363 g
1 serving (12.8 oz)

Calories 590
From fat 466

Amount	% Daily Value*	Amount	% Daily Value*
Total Fat 52.6g	81%	**Total Carbohydrates** 10g	3%
Saturated 29.9g	149%	Dietary Fiber 2g	9%
Trans Fat 1.3g		Sugars 6g	
Cholesterol 458mg	153%	**Protein** 22g	43%
Sodium 513mg	21%		
Calcium 30% • **Iron** 13%		**Vitamin A** 45% • **Vitamin C** 95%	

* Percent Daily Values are based on 2000 calorie diet. Your Daily Values may be higher or lower depending on your calorie needs.

INSTRUCTIONS:

1. Preheat the oven to 375 F.
2. Melt 1 tbsp of butter in a small frying pan under medium heat.
3. Add the sliced white mushrooms to the frying pan and sauté for 5 minutes.
4. Add the garlic, white onions, and bell peppers Cook for an additional 2 to 3 minutes while stirring.
5. Add the sliced zucchini and cook unit wilted.
6. In a medium-sized, whisk together the eggs and heavy cream until airy.
7. Prepare a small springform pan by brushing the bottom and sides with the remaining butter.
8. Pour the whisked egg into the springform pan and drop in the cooked vegetables. Add shredded cheddar to the top.
9. Bake in the oven for 25 to 30 minutes. Allow to cool before serving.

Asparagus and Tofu Stir Fry

INGREDIENTS	Protein	Fat	Carbs
5 spears asparagus	1.32 g	0.07 g	2.33 g
1 1/4 cup broccoli, chopped	1.59 g	0.25 g	1.43 g
1 tsp sesame seeds	0.55 g	1.65 g	0.32 g
1 tbsp sesame oil	0 g	13.6 g	0 g
1 1/2 tbsp olive oil	0 g	20.3 g	0 g
1/4 tbsp garlic, chopped	0.13 g	0.01 g	0.69 g
1 tbsp soy sauce	1.29 g	0.04 g	0.79 g
1/4 cup peanuts, chopped	8.18 g	16.73 g	6.75 g
1 cup firm tofu, cubed	20.64 g	10.5 g	4.26 g

Nutrition Facts

Amount per 441 g
1 serving (15.6 oz)

Calories 663
From fat 495

	Amount	% Daily Value*	Amount	% Daily Value*
	Total Fat 56.4g	87%	Total Carbohydrates 17g	6%
	Saturated 8.7g	43%	Dietary Fiber 8g	32%
	Trans Fat 0g		Sugars 4g	
	Cholesterol 0mg	0%	Protein 34g	67%
	Sodium 760mg	32%		
	Calcium 60% • Iron 42%		Vitamin A 35% • Vitamin C 25%	

* Percent Daily Values are based on 2000 calorie diet. Your Daily Values may be higher or lower depending on your calorie needs.

INSTRUCTIONS:

1. Preheat the oven to 450 F.
2. In a small bowl, toss the tofu with olive oil, salt, and pepper. Place the tofu cubes on a baking tray, taking care that they don't touch each other.
3. Bake the tofu in the oven for 20 to 25 minutes, or until the outer surface of the cubes are firm.
4. Preheat the remaining olive oil and sesame oil in a large frying pan over high heat.
5. Add the chopped peanuts to the pan and cook for 1 to 2 minutes while constantly stirring.

6. Add the cooked tofu and stir in.
7. Add the chopped broccoli and the asparagus. Continue to stir while cooking for about 4 to 5 minutes, or just until the vegetables have started to turn a bright green color.
8. Add the soy sauce and stir. Cook for an additional 1 minute.
9. Sprinkle with sesame seeds and transfer to a bowl.

Serve while hot•

Roasted Cauliflower Soup

INGREDIENTS	Protein	Fat	Carbs
1 1/4 cup cauliflower, chopped	2.57 g	0.37 g	6.65 g
1 3/4 cup butter	0.21 g	20.2 g	0.01 g
1/2 tbsp white onion, chopped	0.06 g	0.01 g	0.47 g
1/4 cup heavy cream	0.62 g	11.1 g	0.84 g
1/4 cup cream cheese	6.88 g	39.72 g	4.72 g
1/2 cup vegetable broth	0 g	0 g	1.5 g
1/4 tbsp onion leeks, chopped	0.12 g	0.02 g	1.13 g
1/2 tbsp olive oil	0 g	6.8 g	0 g

Nutrition Facts

Amount per 442 g
1 serving (15.6 oz)

Calories 785
From fat 688

Amount	% Daily Value*	Amount	% Daily Value*
Total Fat 78.2g	120%	Total Carbohydrates 15g	5%
Saturated 43.2g	216%	Dietary Fiber 3g	12%
Trans Fat 0.8g		Sugars 9g	
Cholesterol 222mg	74%	Protein 10g	21%
Sodium 1107mg	46%		
Calcium 18% • Iron 7%		Vitamin A 60% • Vitamin C 110%	

* Percent Daily Values are based on 2000 calorie diet. Your Daily Values may be higher or lower depending on your calorie needs.

<u>**INSTRUCTIONS:**</u>

1. Preheat the oven to 400 F.
2. Spread the chopped cauliflower on a large baking tray and drizzle with the olive oil.
3. Roast cauliflower in the oven for 20 minutes, stirring just once midway.
4. Melt the butter in a medium-sized pot over medium heat. Add the chopped white onion and cook until soft.
5. Add the vegetable broth and the roasted cauliflower to the pot and allow to boil.
6. While still hot, stir in the heavy cream and the cream cheese. Stir thoroughly.
7. Transfer the contents of the pot into a food processor and pulse until smooth.
8. Sprinkle with chopped onion leeks before serving. Serve while hot.

DAY 4

BREAKFAST	Yogurt Bowl with Nuts and Seeds	513
LUNCH	High-Protein Cauliflower Flatbread	605
DINNER	Broccoli and Mushroom in Cheese Sauce	754

Yogurt Bowl with Nuts and Seeds

INGREDIENTS	Protein	Fat	Carbs
3/4 cup coconut milk	3.42 g	36. 15 g	4.76 g
1 cup Greek yogurt	10.19 g	0.39 g	3.6 g

INGREDIENTS	Protein	Fat	Carbs
1 tbsp protein powder	5.03 g	1.89 g	2.04 g
1tbsp pecans, chopped	0.63 g	5.19 g	0.9 g
1/2 tbsp sunflower seeds	0.91 g	2.26 g	0.88 g

<table>
<tr><td colspan="2">Nutrition Facts
Amount per 292 g
1 serving (10.3 oz)
Calories 513
From fat 385</td><td>Amount</td><td>% Daily Value*</td><td>Amount</td><td>% Daily Value*</td></tr>
<tr><td colspan="2"></td><td colspan="2">Total Fat 45.9g   71%</td><td colspan="2">Total Carbohydrates 12g   4%</td></tr>
<tr><td colspan="2"></td><td colspan="2">Saturated 33g   165%</td><td colspan="2">Dietary Fiber 2g   7%</td></tr>
<tr><td colspan="2"></td><td colspan="2">Trans Fat 0g</td><td colspan="2">Sugars 4g</td></tr>
<tr><td colspan="2"></td><td colspan="2">Cholesterol 7mg   2%</td><td colspan="2">Protein 20g   40%</td></tr>
<tr><td colspan="2"></td><td colspan="2">Sodium 122mg   5%</td><td colspan="2"></td></tr>
<tr><td colspan="2"></td><td colspan="2">Calcium 20% • Iron 39%</td><td colspan="2">Vitamin A 6% • Vitamin C 9%</td></tr>
<tr><td colspan="6">* Percent Daily Values are based on 2000 calorie diet. Your Daily Values may be higher or lower depending on your calorie needs.</td></tr>
</table>

INSTRUCTIONS:

1. Combine the coconut milk, yogurt, and protein powder in a blender. Blend until smooth.
2. Transfer the contents of the blender into a bowl and add the pecans and sunflower seeds.
3. The yogurt bowl is best served slightly chilled.

High-Protein Cauliflower Flatbread

INGREDIENTS	Protein	Fat	Carbs
2 cups cauliflower, chopped	4.11 g	0.6 g	10.64 g
2 eggs	11.05 g	8.37 g	0.63 g
1/2 tbsp garlic, chopped	0.27 g	0.02 g	1.42 g
2 tbsp butter	0.24 g	23.04 g	0.02 g

1/2 cup mozzarella, shredded	12.42 g	12.52 g	1.23 g
1/2 tbsp parsley	0.06 g	0.02 g	0.12 g
1/2 tsp oregano	0.05 g	0.02 g	0.34 g
1 tbsp protein powder	5.03 g	1.89 g	2.04 g

Nutrition Facts

Amount per 404 g
1 serving (14.3 oz)

Calories 605
From fat 410

Amount	% Daily Value*	Amount	% Daily Value*
Total Fat 46.5g	71%	**Total Carbohydrates** 16g	5%
Saturated 25.2g	126%	Dietary Fiber 5g	22%
Trans Fat 1g		Sugars 6g	
Cholesterol 435mg	145%	**Protein** 33g	66%
Sodium 761mg	32%		
Calcium 46% • **Iron** 22%		**Vitamin A** 40% • **Vitamin C** 184%	

* Percent Daily Values are based on 2000 calorie diet. Your Daily Values may be higher or lower depending on your calorie needs.

INSTRUCTIONS:

1. Preheat the oven to 400 F.
2. Place the chopped cauliflower in a steamer and cook for 10 minutes or until tender.
3. Transfer the cooked cauliflower into a food processor. Pulse until very fine.
4. Wrap the ground cauliflower with a kitchen tower and squeeze to remove moisture. Allow the cauliflower to rest for 10 minutes before repeating the squeezing process. Repeat this process one more time.
5. Combine the ground cauliflower, butter, eggs, protein powder, garlic, oregano, and parsley in a large bowl. Mix until thoroughly combined.
6. Transfer the dough mixture into a baking tray lined with parchment paper. Pat the dough flat up to about a quarter of an inch thickness.
7. Bake in the oven for 30 to 40 minutes, or until the top of the bread has turned golden brown.
8. Remove from the oven. Cool for about 10 minutes before serving. Serve while warm.

Broccoli and Mushroom in Cheese Sauce

INGREDIENTS	Protein	Fat	Carbs
2 cups white mushrooms, sliced	4.33 g	0.48 g	4.56 g
3 cups broccoli, chopped	3.8 g	0.59 g	3.42 g
1/2 tbsp garlic, chopped	0.27 g	0.02 g	1.42 g
3/4 cup heavy cream	1.85 g	33.3 g	2.51 g
1/2 cup cheddar, grated	15.87 g	22.32 g	0.88 g
1/2 tbsp olive oil	0 g	6.8 g	0 g
1/2 tbsp butter	0.06 g	5.76 g	0 g
1 tbsp basil, chopped	0.09 g	0.02 g	0.07 g

Nutrition Facts

Amount per 437 g
1 serving (15.4 oz)

Calories 754
From fat 614

Amount	% Daily Value*	Amount	% Daily Value*
Total Fat 69.3g	107%	Total Carbohydrates 13g	4%
Saturated 38.2g	191%	Dietary Fiber 5g	19%
Trans Fat 1g		Sugars 6g	
Cholesterol 206mg	69%	Protein 26g	53%
Sodium 552mg	23%		
Calcium 65% • Iron 20%		Vitamin A 109% • Vitamin C 49%	

* Percent Daily Values are based on 2000 calorie diet. Your Daily Values may be higher or lower depending on your calorie needs.

INSTRUCTIONS:

1. In a food processor, combine the heavy cream, butter, cheddar, basil, and garlic. Blend until smooth and set aside.
2. In a large frying pan, preheat the olive oil over high heat.
3. Add the white mushrooms and cook for 8 to 10 minutes, or until slightly brown.

4. Add the broccoli and cook for an additional 3 to 4 minutes, or until the broccoli has turned bright green.
5. Remove the mushrooms and broccoli from the heat and combine with the cheese sauce. Mix until well-combined.
6. Serve while hot.

DAY 5

BREAKFAST	Overnight Coconut Chia Pudding	593
LUNCH	Cheesy Cream of Mushroom Soup	817
DINNER	Zucchini and Cabbage Salad	536

Overnight Coconut Chia Pudding

INGREDIENTS	Protein	Fat	Carbs
3/4 cup coconut milk	3.42 g	36.15 g	4.76 g
1/4 tbsp chia seeds	1.32 g	2.46 g	3.37 g
1/2 tbsp coconut oil	0 g	6.8 g	0 g
1/4 tbsp desiccated coconut	0.42 g	5.53 g	1.72 g
1/2 tbsp pecans, ground	0.31 g	2.56 g	0.44 g
1 tbsp protein powder	5.03 g	1.89 g	2.04 g
1/4 cup milk	1.92 g	1.99 g	2.92 g

<table>
<tr><td rowspan="6">Nutrition Facts

Amount per 268 g
1 serving (9.4 oz)

Calories 593
From fat 484</td><td>Amount</td><td>% Daily Value*</td><td>Amount</td><td>% Daily Value*</td></tr>
<tr><td>Total Fat 57.4g</td><td>88%</td><td>Total Carbohydrates 15g</td><td>5%</td></tr>
<tr><td>Saturated 44.7g</td><td>223%</td><td>Dietary Fiber 4g</td><td>16%</td></tr>
<tr><td>Trans Fat 0g</td><td></td><td>Sugars 4g</td><td></td></tr>
<tr><td>Cholesterol 8mg</td><td>3%</td><td>Protein 12g</td><td>25%</td></tr>
<tr><td>Sodium 102mg</td><td>4%</td><td></td><td></td></tr>
<tr><td colspan="5">Calcium 21% • Iron 42%   Vitamin A 8% • Vitamin C 9%</td></tr>
<tr><td colspan="5">* Percent Daily Values are based on 2000 calorie diet. Your Daily Values may be higher or lower depending on your calorie needs.</td></tr>
</table>

INSTRUCTIONS:

1. In a blender, combine the milk, coconut milk, coconut oil, and protein powder. Blend until smooth.
2. Transfer the blended ingredients into a container that can be covered. Add the chia seeds and stir thoroughly.
3. Cover the container and place in the refrigerator overnight.
4. Add the desiccated coconut and ground pecans right before serving.
5. Serve while still slightly chilled.

Cheesy Cream of Mushroom Soup

INGREDIENTS	Protein	Fat	Carbs
1 1/2 cup white mushroom, sliced	4.45 g	0.49 g	4.69 g
1 cup heavy cream	2.46 g	44.4 g	3.35 g
1/4 cup vegetable broth	0 g	0 g	0.75 g
2 tbsp butter	0.24 g	23.04 g	0.02 g
1/4 tbsp garlic, chopped	0.13 g	0.01 g	0.69 g
1/2 tbsp white onion, chopped	0.06 g	0.01 g	0.47 g

INGREDIENTS	Protein	Fat	Carbs
1 tbsp olive oil	0 g	13.5 g	0 g
1/3 cup mozzarella, shredded	8.97 g	0 g	0.99 g

<table>
<tr><td colspan="3">Nutrition Facts</td><td>Amount</td><td>% Daily Value*</td><td>Amount</td><td>% Daily Value*</td></tr>
<tr><td colspan="3">Amount per 400 g</td><td>Total Fat 81.4g</td><td>125%</td><td>Total Carbohydrates 11g</td><td>4%</td></tr>
<tr><td colspan="3">1 serving (14.1 oz)</td><td>Saturated 44.2g</td><td>221%</td><td>Dietary Fiber 2g</td><td>8%</td></tr>
<tr><td colspan="3"></td><td>Trans Fat 0.9g</td><td></td><td>Sugars 7g</td><td></td></tr>
<tr><td colspan="3">Calories 817</td><td>Cholesterol 231mg</td><td>77%</td><td>Protein 16g</td><td>33%</td></tr>
<tr><td colspan="3">From fat 716</td><td>Sodium 682mg</td><td>28%</td><td></td><td></td></tr>
<tr><td colspan="3"></td><td>Calcium 37% • Iron</td><td>5%</td><td>Vitamin A 55% • Vitamin C</td><td>8%</td></tr>
</table>

* Percent Daily Values are based on 2000 calorie diet. Your Daily Values may be higher or lower depending on your calorie needs.

INSTRUCTIONS:

1. In a large saucepan, combine the butter and olive oil. Preheat over medium heat.
2. Add the white onions and garlic. Cook while stirring until the onions are soft, about 4 to 5 minutes.
3. Add the white mushrooms. Continue cooking while stirring for about 9 to 10 minutes, or until the mushrooms have become slightly brown.
4. Add the vegetable broth and heavy cream. Continue stirring until the soup has boiled.
5. Reduce the heat to a simmer and cook for an additional 10 minutes.
6. Ladle the soup into a bowl and top with shredded mozzarella. Serve while hot.

Zucchini and Cabbage Salad

INGREDIENTS	Protein	Fat	Carbs
2 cups cabbage, shredded	2.28 g	0.18 g	10.32 g

Ingredient			
1 large zucchini, sliced	0.43 g	0.06 g	0.5 g
1/2 tbsp sesame seeds	0.41 g	1.22 g	0.23 g
3/4 tbsp walnuts, ground	1.42 g	3.5 g	0.57 g
1/2 tbsp sesame oil	0 g	6.8 g	0 g
1 1/2 tbsp olive oil	0 g	20.3 g	0 g
1/2 tbsp cider vinegar	0 g	0 g	0.07 g
1/2 cup feta cheese, crumbled	10.66 g	15.96 g	3.07 g

Nutrition Facts

Amount per 312 g
1 serving (11 oz)

Calories 536
From fat 421

Amount	% Daily Value*	Amount	% Daily Value*
Total Fat 48g	74%	**Total Carbohydrates** 15g	5%
Saturated 15.4g	77%	Dietary Fiber 5g	21%
Trans Fat 0g		Sugars 9g	
Cholesterol 67mg	22%	**Protein** 15g	30%
Sodium 722mg	30%		
Calcium 45% • **Iron** 11%		**Vitamin A** 11% • **Vitamin C** 118%	

* Percent Daily Values are based on 2000 calorie diet. Your Daily Values may be higher or lower depending on your calorie needs.

INSTRUCTIONS:

1. Combine the sesame seeds and ground walnuts in a dry frying pan and toast over low heat until fragrant.
2. In a large bowl, combine the sliced zucchini, cabbage, sesame seeds, and walnuts. Toss lightly.
3. In a separate bowl, whisk together the olive oil, sesame oil, and cider vinegar. Season with salt and pepper if desired.
4. Add the dressing to the salat and toss well.
5. Sprinkle the feta cheese on top of the salad and serve.

DAY 6

BREAKFAST	Spinach Mushroom Frittata	559
LUNCH	Keto Summer Salad	668
DINNER	Asian Egg Drop Soup	609

Spinach Mushroom Frittata

INGREDIENTS	Protein	Fat	Carbs
2 eggs	11.05 g	8.37 g	0.63 g
1/2 cup milk	3.84 g	3.99 g	5.83 g
1 cup spinach	0.86 g	0.12 g	1.09 g
1/2 cup white mushroom, sliced	1.08 g	0.12 g	1.14 g
1/2 tbsp white onion, chopped	0.06 g	0.01 g	0.47 g
1/2 tbsp garlic, chopped	0.27 g	0.02 g	1.42 g
1/4 cup cheddar, shredded	6.8 g	9.57 g	0.38 g
1 tbsp butter	0.12 g	11.52 g	0.01 g
1 tbsp olive oil	0 g	13.5 g	0 g

Nutrition Facts

Amount per 340 g
1 serving (12 oz)

Calories 559
From fat 420

	Amount	% Daily Value*	Amount	% Daily Value*
Total Fat	47.2g	73%	Total Carbohydrates 11g	4%
Saturated	19.7g	99%	Dietary Fiber 1g	5%
Trans Fat	0.8g		Sugars 8g	
Cholesterol	399mg	133%	Protein 24g	48%
Sodium	478mg	20%		
Calcium	42% • Iron 15%		Vitamin A 82% • Vitamin C	18%

* Percent Daily Values are based on 2000 calorie diet. Your Daily Values may be higher or lower depending on your calorie needs.

<u>**INSTRUCTIONS:**</u>

1. In a large pan, melt the butter over medium heat. Add the olive oil.
2. Add the white onion and garlic to the pan and cook until the onion has become soft, about 3 to 4 minutes.
3. Add the white mushroom and cook for an additional 8 to 10 minutes, or until the mushrooms has turned light brown.
4. Add the spinach to the pan and mix well. Cook for an additional 2 minutes. Set aside.
5. In a large bowl, whisk together the 2 eggs, butter, and milk.
6. Transfer the egg mixture into a deep pan. Add the cooked mushrooms and spinach and stir together.
7. Cook the egg mixture over low heat for 9 to 10 minutes, or until the top layer has set. A minute before the eggs are done, sprinkle the shredded cheddar over the top.
8. Allow to cool for 5 minutes before serving.

Keto Summer Salad

INGREDIENTS	Protein	Fat	Carbs
3 cups romaine lettuce, shredded	1.73 g	0.42 g	4.64 g
1/2 cup avocado, cubed	1.5 g	11 g	6.4 g
1/2 tbsp red onion, chopped	0.06 g	0.01 g	0.47 g
1/2 tbsp cilantro, chopped	0.01 g	0 g	0.02 g
1 tbsp olive oil	0 g	13.5 g	0 g
1 tbsp lemon juice	0.05 g	0.04 g	1.06 g
1/2 cup cheddar, diced	15.87 g	22.32 g	0.88 g

| 1/4 cup walnuts, ground | 3.05 g | 13.04 g | 2.74 g |

Nutrition Facts

Amount per 336 g
1 serving (11.9 oz)

Calories 668
From fat 525

	Amount	% Daily Value*	Amount	% Daily Value*
Total Fat 60.3g		93%	**Total Carbohydrates** 16g	5%
Saturated 17.5g		88%	Dietary Fiber 10g	38%
Trans Fat 0.8g			Sugars 3g	
Cholesterol 67mg		22%	**Protein** 22g	45%
Sodium 443mg		18%		
Calcium 52% • **Iron** 14%			**Vitamin A** 262% • **Vitamin C** 33%	

* Percent Daily Values are based on 2000 calorie diet. Your Daily Values may be higher or lower depending on your calorie needs.

INSTRUCTIONS:

1. In a large bowl, combine the lettuce, avocado, red onion, and cilantro.
2. In a smaller bowl, whisk together the lemon juice and olive oil. Drizzle over the salad.
3. Sprinkle the cheddar and walnuts over the salad. Season with salt and pepper if desired. Toss well.
4. Serve immediately.

Asian Egg Drop Soup

INGREDIENTS	Protein	Fat	Carbs
1 1/2 cup vegetable broth	0 g	0 g	4.51 g
1/2 cup coconut milk	2.28 g	24.1 g	3.18 g
1 egg	5.53 g	4.18 g	0.32 g
1 tbsp sesame oil	0 g	13.6 g	0 g
1/2 tbsp ginger, sliced	0.05 g	0.02 g	0.53 g
1 tbsp butter	0.12 g	11.52 g	0.01 g
1/2 tbsp lemon juice	0.03 g	0.02 g	0.52 g
1/2 tbsp fish sauce	0.46 g	0 g	0.33 g

| 1/2 tbsp green onion, sliced | 0.03 g | 0.01 g | 0.17 g |
| 1/2 cup soft tofu, cubes | 8.12 g | 4.58 g | 2.23 g |

Nutrition Facts

Amount per 684 g
1 serving (24.1 oz)

Calories 609
From fat 500

Amount	% Daily Value*	Amount	% Daily Value*
Total Fat 58g	89%	**Total Carbohydrates** 12g	4%
Saturated 32.6g	163%	Dietary Fiber 0g	2%
Trans Fat 0.5g		Sugars 5g	
Cholesterol 194mg	65%	**Protein** 17g	33%
Sodium 2296mg	96%		
Calcium 19% • **Iron** 33%		**Vitamin A** 29% • **Vitamin C** 8%	

* Percent Daily Values are based on 2000 calorie diet. Your Daily Values may be higher or lower depending on your calorie needs.

INSTRUCTIONS:

1. In a small pot, bring the vegetable broth to a boil and add the ginger. Simmer for 15 minutes.
2. Remove the ginger from the broth and discard.
3. To the broth, stir in the coconut milk, lemon juice, fish sauce, and sesame oil. Heat until boiling.
4. While the broth is boiling, drop in the cubes of soft tofu. Allow the broth to simmer for an additional 15 minutes.
5. In a small bowl, whisk together the egg and butter.
6. Slowly pour in the whisked egg to the broth while stirring.
7. Turn off the heat and ladle the soup into a serving bowl. Garnish with the green onions before serving.

DAY 7

BREAKFAST	Curried Tofu Scramble with Mushrooms	543
LUNCH	Greek-Style Keto Salad	638
DINNER	Spicy Cauliflower Soup	643

Curried Tofu Scramble with Mushrooms

INGREDIENTS	Protein	Fat	Carbs
2 cups firm tofu, diced	23.74 g	13.99 g	4.8 g
1 cup white mushroom, sliced	2.97 g	0.33 g	3.13 g
1 sweet red pepper, chopped	1.18 g	0.36 g	7.18 g
1/2 cup spinach	0.43 g	0.06 g	0.54 g
1 tbsp curry powder	0.9 g	0.88 g	3.52 g
1/2 tbsp fish sauce	0.46 g	0 g	0.33 g
1 tbsp sesame oil	0 g	13.6 g	0 g
1 tbsp olive oil	0 g	13.5 g	0 g

Nutrition Facts

Amount per 512 g
1 serving (18.1 oz)

Calories 543
From fat 371

	Amount	% Daily Value*		Amount	% Daily Value*
Total Fat 42.7g		66%	**Total Carbohydrates** 19g		6%
Saturated 5.3g		26%	Dietary Fiber 8g		32%
Trans Fat 0g			Sugars 9g		
Cholesterol 0mg		0%	**Protein** 30g		59%
Sodium 751mg		31%			
Calcium 48% • **Iron** 40%			**Vitamin A** 103% • **Vitamin C** 266%		

* Percent Daily Values are based on 2000 calorie diet. Your Daily Values may be higher or lower depending on your calorie needs.

INSTRUCTIONS:

1. In a large pan, preheat the sesame oil and olive oil over medium heat.
2. Add the white mushroom and cook while continuously stirring for 9 to 10 minutes, or until the mushroom has turned light brown.
3. Add the diced tofu. Continue to stir the contents of the pan while cooking. It is fine to let some of the tofu crumble. Cook for 9 to 10 minutes or until the tofu has become firm.

4. Add the curry powder and fish sauce. Stir well, ensuring that all of the tofu pieces have been coated with the curry powder.
5. Add the red pepper and spinach. Stir while cooking for an additional 3 to 4 minutes.
6. Transfer to a plate and serve while hot.

Greek-Style Keto Salad

INGREDIENTS	Protein	Fat	Carbs
2 cups romaine lettuce, shredded	1.16 g	0.28 g	3.09 g
1/4 cup red onion, sliced	0.32 g	0.03 g	2.69 g
1/2 cup cucumber, sliced	0.35 g	0.1 g	1.29 g
1/2 tbsp olives, sliced	0.04 g	0.45 g	0.26 g
1 tbsp walnuts, ground	1.88 g	4.63 g	0.75 g
3/4 cup feta cheese, crumbled	15.99 g	23.94 g	4.6 g
2 tbsp olive oil	0 g	27 g	0 g
1 tbsp balsamic vinegar	0.08 g	0 g	2.72

Nutrition Facts

Amount per 350 g
1 serving (12.3 oz)

Calories 638
From fat 495

Amount	% Daily Value*	Amount	% Daily Value*
Total Fat 56.4g	87%	Total Carbohydrates 15g	5%
Saturated 20.9g	105%	Dietary Fiber 4g	14%
Trans Fat 0g		Sugars 10g	
Cholesterol 100mg	33%	Protein 20g	40%
Sodium 1077mg	45%		
Calcium 61% • Iron 14%		Vitamin A 175% • Vitamin C 13%	

* Percent Daily Values are based on 2000 calorie diet. Your Daily Values may be higher or lower depending on your calorie needs.

<u>**INSTRUCTIONS:**</u>

1. In a large bowl, combine the lettuce, red onion, cucumber, and olives.
2. In a separate smaller bowl, whisk together the olive oil and balsamic vinegar. Drizzle the dressing over the salad and toss well.
3. Sprinkle the ground walnuts and feta cheese over the salad right before serving.

Spicy Cauliflower Soup

INGREDIENTS	Protein	Fat	Carbs
1/2 cup cauliflower, chopped	1.03 g	0.15 g	2.66 g
1/2 cup coconut milk	2.28 g	24.1 g	3.18 g
1 tbsp white onion, chopped	0.06 g	0.01 g	0.47 g
1/2 cup vegetable broth	0 g	0 g	1.5 g
1 1/2 tbsp butter	0.18 g	17.28 g	0.01 g
1 tbsp sesame oil	0 g	13.6 g	0 g
1 tbsp lemon juice	0.05 g	0.04 g	1.06 g
1/2 tbsp green onion, chopped	0.03 g	0.01 g	0.17 g
3/4 cup soft tofu, cubed	12.18 g	6.86 g	3.35 g
1/2 tsp. red chili pepper, chopped	0.42 g	0.1 g	1.98 g

Nutrition Facts	Amount	% Daily Value*	Amount	% Daily Value*
	Total Fat 62.2g	96%	**Total Carbohydrates** 14g	5%
Amount per 551 g	Saturated 35.3g	177%	Dietary Fiber 2g	8%
1 serving (19.4 oz)	Trans Fat 0.7g		Sugars 5g	
	Cholesterol 46mg	15%	**Protein** 16g	32%
Calories 643	**Sodium** 655mg	27%		
From fat 534	**Calcium** 25% • **Iron** 35%		**Vitamin A** 23% • **Vitamin C** 111%	

* Percent Daily Values are based on 2000 calorie diet. Your Daily Values may be higher or lower depending on your calorie needs.

INSTRUCTIONS:

1. In a large saucepan, melt the butter with the sesame oil over medium heat.
2. Add the white onion and the red chili pepper. Cook until the onion is soft, about 3 to 4 minutes.
3. Add the chopped cauliflower and cook for another 3 to 4 minutes.
4. Add the coconut milk and vegetable broth. Heat until boiling and allow to simmer for 10 minutes.
5. Turn off the heat and transfer the contents of the saucepan to a blender. Blend until smooth.
6. Pour the blended soup back into the saucepan and heat to a simmer.
7. Add the tofu cubes and stir. Simmer for another 10 minutes.
8. Turn off the heat and add the lemon juice. Stir well.
9. Put the soup into a serving bowl. Garnish with the green onion before serving.

Other Keto Vegetarian Recipes

Easy Keto Bagels

INGREDIENTS	Protein	Fat	Carbs
1 egg	5.53 g	4.18 g	0.32 g
3/4 cup almond flour	15.08 g	35.6 g	15.37 g
1/2 tbsp baking powder	0 g	0.02 g	1.78 g
1/2 cup mozzarella cheese	17.91 g	0 g	1.98 g
1/4 cup cream cheese	3.44 g	19.86 g	2.36 g
1 tsp sesame seeds	0.55 g	1.65 g	0.32 g
1 tsp poppy seeds	0.5 g	1.16 g	0.79 g
1 tbsp butter	0.12 g	11.52 g	0.01 g

Nutrition Facts

Amount per 253 g
1 serving (8.9 oz)

Calories 891
From fat 635

Amount	% Daily Value*	Amount	% Daily Value*
Total Fat 74g	114%	Total Carbohydrates 23g	8%
Saturated 22.9g	115%	Dietary Fiber 11g	44%
Trans Fat 0.5g		Sugars 6g	
Cholesterol 268mg	89%	Protein 43g	86%
Sodium 791mg	33%		
Calcium 103% • Iron 25%		Vitamin A 33% • Vitamin C 0%	

* Percent Daily Values are based on 2000 calorie diet. Your Daily Values may be higher or lower depending on your calorie needs.

INSTRUCTIONS:
1. Preheat oven to 450 F.
2. In a large bowl, combine the almond flour and baking powder. Whisk together.
3. In a separate glass bowl, combine the mozzarella cheese and cream cheese. Microwave for 30 seconds to 1 minute, or until the cheese has been completely melted. Stir together to combine.
4. Pour the cheese mixture into the bowl with the flour and baking powder.
5. Add the egg.
6. Mix the dough together until thoroughly combined.
7. Divide the dough into four equal portions.
8. Prepare a baking tray by lining it with parchment paper.

9. Form a ball from each portion of the dough and place on the baking tray. Press a hole into the center of each ball to form a bagel shape.
10. Sprinkle each bagel with the sesame seeds and poppy seeds.
11. Bake the bagels in the oven for 20 to 25 minutes, or until golden brown.
12. Remove from the oven and allow to cool for about 10 minutes before serving.

Arugula Salad with Avocado

INGREDIENTS	Protein	Fat	Carbs
3 cups arugula	1.55 g	0.40 g	2.19 g
3/4 cup iceberg lettuce, shredded	0.49 g	0.08 g	1.6 g
1/4 avocado, sliced	1.01 g	7.37 g	4.29 g
1/2 tbsp red onion, chopped	0.06 g	0.01 g	0.47 g
1 tbsp basil, chopped	0.09 g	0.02 g	0.07 g
1/2 cup feta cheese, crumbled	10.66 g	15.96 g	3.07 g
1/2 tbsp balsamic vinegar	0.04 g	0 g	1.36 g
2 tbsp olive oil	0g	27 g	0 g
1/4 cup almonds, slivered	5.71 g	13.48 g	5.82 g

<table>
<tr><td rowspan="2">Nutrition Facts

Amount per 309 g
1 serving (10.9 oz)

Calories 706
From fat 558</td><td colspan="2">Amount   % Daily Value*</td><td colspan="2">Amount   % Daily Value*</td></tr>
<tr><td>Total Fat 64.3g</td><td>99%</td><td>Total Carbohydrates 19g</td><td>6%</td></tr>
<tr><td></td><td>Saturated 17.1g</td><td>85%</td><td>Dietary Fiber 9g</td><td>34%</td></tr>
<tr><td></td><td>Trans Fat 0g</td><td></td><td>Sugars 8g</td><td></td></tr>
<tr><td></td><td>Cholesterol 67mg</td><td>22%</td><td>Protein 20g</td><td>39%</td></tr>
<tr><td></td><td>Sodium 716mg</td><td>30%</td><td></td><td></td></tr>
<tr><td></td><td colspan="2">Calcium 56% • Iron 18%</td><td colspan="2">Vitamin A 45% • Vitamin C 27%</td></tr>
<tr><td></td><td colspan="4">* Percent Daily Values are based on 2000 calorie diet. Your Daily Values may be higher or lower depending on your calorie needs.</td></tr>
</table>

INSTRUCTIONS:

1. In a large mixing bowl, combine the arugula, iceberg lettuce, red onion, and basil.
2. In a smaller bowl, mix the balsamic vinegar and olive oil. Whisk together until well-combined.
3. Drizzle the dressing to the salad.
4. Sprinkle the feta cheese and slivered almond over the top.
5. Toss the salad well until thoroughly combined. Serve immediately.

Keto Hash Browns

INGREDIENTS	Protein	Fat	Carbs
1 1/2 cup cauliflower, chopped	3.08 g	0.45 g	7.98 g
2 eggs	11.05 g	8.37 g	0.63 g
2 tbsp butter	0.24 g	23.04 g	0.02 g
1/2 cup almond flour	10.05 g	23.72 g	10.24 g
1/4 tbsp corn starch	0.24 g	0.12 g	1.93 g
1 tbsp coconut oil	0 g	13.6 g	0 g

<table>
<tr><td rowspan="2">Nutrition Facts

Amount per 341 g
1 serving (12 oz)

Calories 771
From fat 599</td><td>Amount</td><td>% Daily Value*</td><td>Amount</td><td>% Daily Value*</td></tr>
<tr><td colspan="2">
<table>
<tr><td>Total Fat 69.3g</td><td>107%</td></tr>
<tr><td>Saturated 31.1g</td><td>156%</td></tr>
<tr><td>Trans Fat 1g</td><td></td></tr>
<tr><td>Cholesterol 388mg</td><td>129%</td></tr>
<tr><td>Sodium 357mg</td><td>15%</td></tr>
<tr><td>Calcium 22% • Iron 23%</td><td></td></tr>
</table>
</td><td colspan="2">
<table>
<tr><td>Total Carbohydrates 21g</td><td>7%</td></tr>
<tr><td>Dietary Fiber 9g</td><td>37%</td></tr>
<tr><td>Sugars 5g</td><td></td></tr>
<tr><td>Protein 25g</td><td>49%</td></tr>
<tr><td></td><td></td></tr>
<tr><td>Vitamin A 24% • Vitamin C 129%</td><td></td></tr>
</table>
</td></tr>
</table>

* Percent Daily Values are based on 2000 calorie diet. Your Daily Values may be higher or lower depending on your calorie needs.

INSTRUCTIONS:

1. Preheat the oven to 400 F.
2. Cook the chopped cauliflower in a steam for 10 minutes. When tender, place the cooked cauliflower in a food processor and blend until very fine.
3. Wrap the ground cauliflower and squeeze to remove any excess moisture. Let the cauliflower rest for about 5 minutes and repeat this process two more times.
4. In a large bowl, combine the ground cauliflower, almond flour, cornstarch, eggs, and coconut oil. Mix until well-combined.
5. Prepare a baking tray by lining it with parchment paper.
6. Place a portion of the cauliflower mash and shape into an oval shape. Repeat until all of the mash has been used.
7. Place the hash browns in the over and bake for 40 to 45 minutes, or until they have turned golden brown and firm.
8. Flip each hash brown and bake the other side for another 5 minutes.
9. Place some butter on top of each hash brown. Return them to the oven and bake for another five minutes.
10. Remove from the oven and allow to cool before serving

Zoodles in Pesto Sauce

INGREDIENTS	Protein	Fat	Carbs
1 medium zucchini	2.37 g	0.63 g	6.1 g

1/2 cup pesto sauce	12.1 g	68.05 g	4.95 g
1 tbsp lemon juice	0.05 g	0.04 g	1.06 g
1/8 cup feta, crumbled	2.77 g	4.15 g	0.8 g
1/8 cup mozzarella, shredded	4.66 g	0 g	0.51 g
1 tbsp walnuts, ground	1.88 g	4.63 g	0.75 g

Nutrition Facts

Amount per 369 g
1 serving (13 oz)

Calories 820
From fat 674

	Amount	% Daily Value*	Amount	% Daily Value*
Total Fat 77.5g		119%	Total Carbohydrates 14g	5%
Saturated 14.8g		74%	Dietary Fiber 4g	16%
Trans Fat 0g			Sugars 7g	
Cholesterol 40mg		13%	Protein 24g	48%
Sodium 1420mg		59%		
Calcium 57% • Iron 19%			Vitamin A 38% • Vitamin C 77%	

* Percent Daily Values are based on 2000 calorie diet. Your Daily Values may be higher or lower depending on your calorie needs.

INSTRUCTIONS:

1. Cut the zucchini into thin strands using a spiralizer
2. Squeeze out as much moisture as possible form the zucchini noodle using a kitchen towel. Set aside.
3. In a medium-sized microwave-safe bowl, combine the parmesan sauce, feta cheese, and mozzarella cheese. Microwave on high for 30 seconds or until the cheese has melted. Stir the sauce until well-combined.
4. In a large bowl, combine the zucchini noodles and the warm pesto sauce. Drizzle lemon juice and sprinkle the walnuts on top.
5. Toss together until all the zucchini noodles have been coated with the sauce. Serve immediately.

Zoodles in Alfredo Sauce

INGREDIENTS	Protein	Fat	Carbs
1 medium zucchini	2.37 g	0.63 g	6.1 g
1 tbsp butter	0.12 g	11.52 g	0.01 g
1 tbsp olive oil	0 g	13.5 g	0 g
1/2 cup white mushroom, sliced	1.48 g	0.16 g	1.56 g
1 tbsp sour cream	0.42 g	1.27 g	0.85 g
1 cup heavy cream	2.46 g	44.4 g	3.35 g
1 tbsp cheddar cheese, shredded	6.8 g	9.57 g	0.38 g

Nutrition Facts

Amount per 432 g
1 serving (15.2 oz)

Calories 810
From fat 715

Amount	% Daily Value*	Amount	% Daily Value*
Total Fat 81.1g	125%	Total Carbohydrates 12g	4%
Saturated 43.3g	216%	Dietary Fiber 2g	10%
Trans Fat 0.8g		Sugars 9g	
Cholesterol 228mg	76%	Protein 14g	27%
Sodium 347mg	14%		
Calcium 32% • Iron 6%		Vitamin A 57% • Vitamin C 62%	

* Percent Daily Values are based on 2000 calorie diet. Your Daily Values may be higher or lower depending on your calorie needs.

INSTRUCTIONS:

1. Using a spiralizer, cut the zucchini into thin strands.
2. Squeeze out as much water as you can from the zucchini noodles using a clean kitchen towel. Set aside.
3. In a large saucepan, melt the butter with the olive oil over medium heat.
4. Add the white mushroom. Cook for 6 to 7 minutes or until the mushroom has turned light brown.
5. Add the heavy cream, sour cream, and cheddar cheese. Lower the heat to a simmer and cook for an additional 5 minutes.
6. Turn off the heat. Pour the alfredo sauce over the zoodles.

7. Toss the zoodles, making sure that each piece has been covered by the sauce. Serve immediately.

Roasted Tofu in Tahini

INGREDIENTS	Protein	Fat	Carbs
1 cup cauliflower, chopped	2.05 g	0.3 g	5.32 g
1 cup firm tofu, diced	39.77 g	21.97 g	10.76 g
1 tbsp tahini	2.55 g	8.06 g	3.18 g
2 tbsp sesame oil	0 g	27.2 g	0 g
1 tbsp lemon juice	0.05 g	0.04 g	1.06 g
1/2 tbsp sesame seeds	0.82 g	2.45 g	0.47 g
1/2 tbsp sunflower seeds	0.91 g	2.26 g	0.88 g

Nutrition Facts

Amount per 425 g
1 serving (15 oz)

Calories 776
From fat 534

	Amount	% Daily Value*	Amount	% Daily Value*
	Total Fat 62.3g	96%	**Total Carbohydrates** 22g	7%
	Saturated 8.9g	44%	Dietary Fiber 10g	41%
	Trans Fat 0g		Sugars 3g	
	Cholesterol 0mg	0%	**Protein** 46g	92%
	Sodium 87mg	4%		
	Calcium 182% • **Iron** 50%		**Vitamin A** 9% • **Vitamin C** 97%	

* Percent Daily Values are based on 2000 calorie diet. Your Daily Values may be higher or lower depending on your calorie needs.

INSTRUCTIONS:

1. Preheat the oven to 400 F.
2. In a large mixing bowl, toss together the cauliflower, tofu, sesame oil, tahini, sesame seeds, and sunflower seeds. Mix well until thoroughly combined.
3. Line a baking tray with parchment paper. Transfer the contents of the mixing bowl into the baking tray, making sure the distribution is as even as possible.

4. Bake in the oven for 25 to 30 minutes, or until the tofu is firm and the cauliflower is tender.
5. Remove the baking tray from the oven and drizzle with lemon juice.
6. Transfer the contents of the baking tray to a bowl. Toss well before serving.

Mixed Greens and Coconut Smoothie

INGREDIENTS	Protein	Fat	Carbs
3/4 cup coconut milk	3.42 g	36.15 g	4.76 g
1/4 cup heavy cream	0.62 g	11.1 g	0.84 g
1/2 cup spinach	0.43 g	0.06 g	0.54 g
1/2 cup arugula	0.26 g	0.07 g	0.37 g
1/4 cup kale	0.17 g	0.04 g	0.35 g
2 tbsp protein powder	10.06 g	3.77 g	4.07 g
2 tbsp coconut oil	0 g	27.2 g	0 g

Nutrition Facts

Amount per 278 g
1 serving (9.8 oz)

Calories 770
From fat 670

	Amount	% Daily Value*	Amount	% Daily Value*
Total Fat	78.4g	121%	Total Carbohydrates 11g	4%
Saturated	62.9g	314%	Dietary Fiber 2g	9%
Trans Fat	0g		Sugars 2g	
Cholesterol	46mg	15%	Protein 15g	30%
Sodium	122mg	5%		
Calcium	20% • Iron 45%		Vitamin A 61% • Vitamin C	32%

* Percent Daily Values are based on 2000 calorie diet. Your Daily Values may be higher or lower depending on your calorie needs.

INSTRUCTIONS:
1. Combine all the ingredients in a blender. Add 3 to 4 ice cubes.
2. Blend until smooth.
3. Serve while chilled.

Baked Eggs in Avocado Boats

INGREDIENTS	Protein	Fat	Carbs
1 whole avocado	4.02 g	29.47 g	17.15 g
2 eggs	11.05 g	8.37 g	0.63 g
1 tbsp chives, chopped	0.1 g	0.02 g	0.13 g
1 tbsp ready-to-serve salsa	0.28 g	0.03 g	1.21 g
1/2 tbsp sesame seeds	0.82 g	2.45 g	0.47 g
1/2 tbsp avocado oil	0 g	7 g	0 g

Nutrition Facts

Amount per 321 g
1 serving (11.3 oz)

Calories 541
From fat 405

Amount	% Daily Value*	Amount	% Daily Value*
Total Fat 47.3g	73%	Total Carbohydrates 20g	7%
Saturated 8.2g	41%	Dietary Fiber 14g	57%
Trans Fat 0g		Sugars 2g	
Cholesterol 327mg	109%	Protein 16g	33%
Sodium 268mg	11%		
Calcium 8% • Iron 17%		Vitamin A 20% • Vitamin C 37%	

* Percent Daily Values are based on 2000 calorie diet. Your Daily Values may be higher or lower depending on your calorie needs.

INSTRUCTIONS:

1. Preheat the oven to 400 F.
2. Split the avocado in half and lay down each half on a baking tray, skin side down.
3. Crack an egg into each avocado half, taking care not to break the yolk.
4. Drizzle avocado oil and sesame seeds over each avocado boat.
5. Place the baking tray in the oven and bake for about 20 minutes, or until the eggs are no longer runny.
6. Remove the tray from the oven and sprinkle with chives. Allow to cool for 10 minutes before serving.

Cauliflower Grilled Cheese Sandwich

INGREDIENTS	Protein	Fat	Carbs
1 1/2 cup cauliflower, chopped	3.08 g	0.45 g	7.98 g
1 egg	5.53 g	4.18 g	0.32 g
1 tbsp green onion, chopped	0.06 g	0.03 g	0.34 g
1/4 tbsp cornstarch	0.01 g	0 g	1.83 g
1/2 cup almond flour	5.03 g	11.88 g	5.13 g
1 tbsp olive oil	0 g	13.5 g	0 g
1 tbsp butter	0.12 g	11.52 g	0.01 g
1/2 cup cheddar, shredded	13.58 g	19.11 g	0.75 g

Nutrition Facts

Amount per 1 serving (11.3 oz) 321 g

Calories 701
From fat 534

	Amount	% Daily Value*	Amount	% Daily Value*
Total Fat	60.7g	93%	Total Carbohydrates 16g	5%
Saturated	22.6g	113%	Dietary Fiber 6g	25%
Trans Fat	1.2g		Sugars 5g	
Cholesterol	252mg	84%	Protein 27g	55%
Sodium	567mg	24%		
Calcium 51% • Iron 14%			Vitamin A 28% • Vitamin C 130%	

* Percent Daily Values are based on 2000 calorie diet. Your Daily Values may be higher or lower depending on your calorie needs.

INSTRUCTIONS:

1. Cook the chopped cauliflower in a steamer for 10 minutes or until tender.
2. Place the cooked cauliflower in a blender and pulse until you get a fine texture.
3. Squeeze the ground cauliflower between kitchen towels and remove as much moisture as you can. Repeat this process two more times.
4. In a large bowl, combine the ground cauliflower, egg, almond flour, and corn starch. Mix well.

5. Combine the olive oil and butter in a frying pan. Preheat at medium heat.
6. Form the cauliflower mash into two square patties. Fry each patty for about 4 to 5 minutes on each side, or until they are firm.
7. After both patties have been cooked, place the shredded cheddar between them.
8. Place the assembled sandwich back in the frying pan and cook for 3 to 4 minutes or until the cheddar has melted.
9. Serve the grilled cheese sandwich while hot.

Triple Green Salad with Asian Dressing

INGREDIENTS	Protein	Fat	Carbs
2 cups kale, chopped	1.37 g	0.3 g	2.8 g
2 cups arugula, chopped	1.03 g	0.26 g	1.46 g
1/4 cup avocado, cubes	0.75 g	5.5 g	3.2 g
1 tsp ginger, grated	0.04 g	0.02 g	0.36 g
1/2 tbsp sesame oil	0 g	6.8 g	0 g
1 tbsp olive oil	0 g	13.5 g	0 g
1/2 tbsp fish sauce	0.46 g	0 g	0.33 g
1 tbsp lemon juice	0.05 g	0.04 g	1.06 g
1/2 cup walnuts, chopped	4.46 g	19.11 g	4.02 g
1/2 cup feta cheese, crumbled	10.66 g	15.96 g	3.07 g
1/2 tbsp sesame seeds	1.64 g	4.9 g	0.94 g

<table>
<tr><td rowspan="2">Nutrition Facts

Amount per 268 g
1 serving (9.5 oz)

Calories 713
From fat 572</td><td colspan="2">Amount</td><td>% Daily Value*</td><td colspan="2">Amount</td><td>% Daily Value*</td></tr>
<tr><td colspan="2">Total Fat 66.4g</td><td>102%</td><td colspan="2">Total Carbohydrates 17g</td><td>6%</td></tr>
</table>

Saturated 17.4g	87%	Dietary Fiber 7g — 29%
Trans Fat 0g		Sugars 6g
Cholesterol 67mg	22%	**Protein** 20g — 41%
Sodium 1425mg	59%	
Calcium 53% • **Iron** 18%		**Vitamin A** 91% • **Vitamin C** 91%

* Percent Daily Values are based on 2000 calorie diet. Your Daily Values may be higher or lower depending on your calorie needs.

INSTRUCTIONS:

1. In a frying pan, lightly toast the walnuts and sesame seeds over low heat. Set aside.
2. In a large bowl, combine the kale, arugula, and avocado.
3. In another bowl, combine the sesame oil, olive oil, ginger, fish sauce, and lemon juice. Whisk together until well-combined.
4. Drizzle the dressing over the salad.
5. Sprinkle the feta cheese, walnuts, and sesame seeds over the top of the salad.
6. Toss well and serve immediately.

Keto Falafel with Tahini Sauce

INGREDIENTS	Protein	Fat	Carbs
1 1/2 cups cauliflower, chopped	3.08 g	0.45 g	7.98 g
1/4 cup almond flour	5.03 g	11.88 g	5.13 g
1/4 cup peanut flour	5.07 g	3.29 g	4.69 g
2 eggs	11.05 g	8.37 g	0.63 g
1 tbsp garlic chopped	0.54 g	0.04 g	2.81 g
1 tbsp cumin	1.07 g	1.34 g	2.65 g

1 tbsp parsley, chopped	0.11 g	0.03 g	0.24 g
1 tbsp tahini	2.55 g	8.06 g	3.18 g
1 tbsp lemon juice	0.0 5g	0.04 g	1.06 g
2 tbsp olive oil	0 g	27 g	0 g

<table>
<tr><td colspan="5">Nutrition Facts</td></tr>
<tr><td></td><td>Amount</td><td>% Daily Value*</td><td>Amount</td><td>% Daily Value*</td></tr>
<tr><td rowspan="7">Amount per 363 g
1 serving (12.8 oz)

Calories 736
From fat 524</td><td>Total Fat 60.5g</td><td>93%</td><td>Total Carbohydrates 28g</td><td>9%</td></tr>
<tr><td>Saturated 9.3g</td><td>46%</td><td>Dietary Fiber 11g</td><td>44%</td></tr>
<tr><td>Trans Fat 0.1g</td><td></td><td>Sugars 5g</td><td></td></tr>
<tr><td>Cholesterol 327mg</td><td>109%</td><td>Protein 29g</td><td>57%</td></tr>
<tr><td>Sodium 205mg</td><td>9%</td><td></td><td></td></tr>
<tr><td>Calcium 31% • Iron 54%</td><td></td><td>Vitamin A 18% • Vitamin C 153%</td><td></td></tr>
<tr><td colspan="4">* Percent Daily Values are based on 2000 calorie diet. Your Daily Values may be higher or lower depending on your calorie needs.</td></tr>
</table>

INSTRUCTIONS:

1. Place the chopped cauliflower in a food processor. Pulse until you get a very fine texture.
2. Squeeze out excess moisture from the ground cauliflower by pressing between clean kitchen towels. Repeat this process two more times.
3. In a large bowl, combine the ground cauliflower, almond flour, peanut flour, eggs, garlic, cumin, and parsley. Mix well until well-combined.
4. Separate the mash into portions and form balls with approximately 1-inch diameters.
5. In a frying pan, preheat the olive oil over medium heat.
6. Fry the falafels taking care not to crowd the frying pan. Cook each falafel for 7 to 8 minutes while occasionally turning to ensure even cooking.
7. Set aside the cooked falafels.
8. Meanwhile, combine the tahini and lemon sauce in a separate bowl. Whisk together.
9. Top each falafel with the tahini sauce before serving.

Tofu in Cream of Asparagus Soup

INGREDIENTS	Protein	Fat	Carbs
1 cup asparagus	2.95 g	0.16 g	5.2 g
1 1/2 cups silky tofu, diced	24.37 g	13.73 g	6.7 g
1/2 cup coconut milk	2.28 g	24.1 g	3.18 g
1 tbsp spring onion, chopped	0.11 g	0.01 g	0.44 g
1 tbsp lemon juice	0.05 g	0.04 g	1.06 g
1 tbsp coconut oil	0 g	13.6 g	0 g
1/4 tbsp sesame oil	0 g	3.4 g	0 g
1/2 tbsp parsley, chopped	0.06 g	0.02 g	0.12 g
1/2 tbsp cilantro, chopped	0.01 g	0 g	0.02 g

Nutrition Facts

Amount per 660 g
1 serving (23.3 oz)

Calories 630
From fat 466

	Amount	% Daily Value*		Amount	% Daily Value*
Total Fat	55.1g	85%	Total Carbohydrates	17g	6%
Saturated	35.7g	178%	Dietary Fiber	4g	15%
Trans Fat	0g		Sugars	6g	
Cholesterol	0mg	0%	Protein	30g	60%
Sodium	50mg	2%			
Calcium	47% • Iron	61%	Vitamin A	26% • Vitamin C	32%

* Percent Daily Values are based on 2000 calorie diet. Your Daily Values may be higher or lower depending on your calorie needs.

INSTRUCTIONS:

1. In a large saucepan, preheat the coconut oil and sesame oil over medium heat.
2. Add the spring onion and asparagus. Cook for 4 to 5 minutes, or until the asparagus has turned a bright green.
3. Add the coconut milk, parsley, and cilantro. Allow to boil. Turn down the heat to a simmer and cook for an additional 10 minutes.

4. Transfer the soup into a blender. Blend until smooth.
5. Return the blended soup to the saucepan and bring to a boil.
6. Add the diced tofu and cook for an additional 10 minutes.
7. Turn off the heat and add the lemon juice. Stir well and serve while hot.

Egg Salad

INGREDIENTS	Protein	Fat	Carbs
2 eggs	11.05 g	8.37 g	0.63 g
3/4 cup avocado, cubes	2.25 g	16.49 g	9.6 g
1/4 cup mayonnaise	0.53 g	41.17 g	0.31 g
1/2 tbsp lemon juice	0.03 g	0.02 g	0.52 g
12 tbsp mustard	0.29 g	0.26 g	0.45 g
1/2 tbsp parsley, chopped	0.06 g	0.02 g	0.12 g

Nutrition Facts

Amount per 273 g
1 serving (9.6 oz)

Calories 687
From fat 586

Amount	% Daily Value*	Amount	% Daily Value*
Total Fat 66.3g	102%	Total Carbohydrates 12g	4%
Saturated 11.6g	58%	Dietary Fiber 8g	32%
Trans Fat 0.1g		Sugars 2g	
Cholesterol 350mg	117%	Protein 14g	28%
Sodium 569mg	24%		
Calcium 8% • Iron 14%		Vitamin A 17% • Vitamin C 28%	

* Percent Daily Values are based on 2000 calorie diet. Your Daily Values may be higher or lower depending on your calorie needs.

INSTRUCTIONS:
1. Boil the eggs for 10 to 15 minutes. Make sure that they are firm after cooking.
2. Run the eggs under cold water and peel the shells.
3. Chop the eggs roughly into small pieces and set aside.
4. Mash the avocado. Set aside.

5. In a large bowl, combine the eggs, mashed avocado, mayonnaise, mustard, lemon, and parsley.
6. Chill the salad for at least an hour before serving.\

Keto Mushroom Pizza

INGREDIENTS	Protein	Fat	Carbs
1 1/2 cups cauliflower	3.08 g	0.45 g	7.98 g
1/4 cup almond flour	5.03 g	11.88 g	5.13 g
2 eggs	11.05 g	8.37 g	0.63 g
1/2 tsp garlic powder	0.26 g	0.01 g	1.16 g
1/2 tsp oregano	0.08 g	0.04 g	0.62 g
1/2 cup white mushroom sliced	2.22 g	0.24 g	2.35 g
1 1/2 tbsp ready-to-serve salsa	0.042 g	0.05 g	1.81 g
1 cup arugula	0.52 g	0.13 g	0.73 g
2 tbsp olive oil	0 g	27 g	0 g

Nutrition Facts

Amount per 421 g
1 serving (14.8 oz)

Calories 579
From fat 421

	Amount	% Daily Value*	Amount	% Daily Value*
Total Fat	48.2g	74%	Total Carbohydrates 20g	7%
Saturated	7.7g	38%	Dietary Fiber 8g	33%
Trans Fat	0.1g		Sugars 7g	
Cholesterol	327mg	109%	Protein 23g	45%
Sodium	374mg	16%		
Calcium 21% • Iron 25%			Vitamin A 22% • Vitamin C 137%	

* Percent Daily Values are based on 2000 calorie diet. Your Daily Values may be higher or lower depending on your calorie needs.

INSTRUCTIONS:
1. Preheat oven to 375 F.
2. Cook the chopped cauliflower in a steamer for 10 minutes, or until tender.
3. Wrap the cooked cauliflower with a kitchen towel and squeeze out as much moisture as possible. Repeat this process two more times.

4. In a large bowl, combine the ground cauliflower, almond flour, eggs, and garlic powder. Mix until well-combined.
5. Line a baking tray with parchment paper. Place the dough on the baking tray and form into a round pizza shape.
6. Bake in the oven for 10 minutes or until firm.
7. Remove the crust from oven and drizzle with olive oil.
8. Apply the salsa evenly to the top of the pizza and scatter the slices of white mushroom.
9. Place the pizza back in the oven and bake for an additional 10 minutes.
10. Remove the pizza from the oven and allow to cool. Top with arugula right before serving.

High-Protein Spinach Smoothie

INGREDIENTS	Protein	Fat	Carbs
1 cup coconut milk	4.57 g	48.21 g	6.35 g
1 cup spinach	0.86 g	0.12 g	1.09 g
1/2 cup cucumber, sliced	0.35 g	0.1 g	1.29 g
1 tsp coconut oil	0 g	4.5 g	0 g
2 tbsp protein powder	10.06 g	3.77 g	4.07 g
1 tsp vanilla extract	0 g	0 g	0.53 g

Nutrition Facts

Amount per 346 g
1 serving (12.2 oz)

Calories 601
From fat 478

	Amount	% Daily Value*	Amount	% Daily Value*
	Total Fat 56.7g	87%	**Total Carbohydrates** 13g	4%
	Saturated 47g	235%	Dietary Fiber 3g	10%
	Trans Fat 0g		Sugars 3g	
	Cholesterol 5mg	2%	**Protein** 16g	32%
	Sodium 127mg	5%		
	Calcium 19% • **Iron** 57%		**Vitamin A** 68% • **Vitamin C** 32%	

* Percent Daily Values are based on 2000 calorie diet. Your Daily Values may be higher or lower depending on your calorie needs.

INSTRUCTIONS:
1. Combine all the ingredients in a blender. Add 5 to 6 ice cubes.

2. Blend until smooth.
3. Serve while chilled.

Cream of Cauliflower Soup

INGREDIENTS	Protein	Fat	Carbs
1 1/2 cups cauliflower	3.08 g	0.45 g	7.98 g
3/4 cup heavy cream	1.85 g	33.3 g	2.51 g
3/4 cup vegetable broth	0 g	0 g	2.26 g
1 tbsp white onion, chopped	0.11 g	0.01 g	0.93 g
1/2 tbsp chives, chopped	0.05 g	0.01 g	0.07 g
2 tbsp butter	0.24 g	23.04 g	0.02 g
1/2 cup white mushrooms	1.48 g	0.16 g	1.56 g
3/4 cup feta cheese, crumbled	15.99 g	23.94 g	4.6 g

Nutrition Facts

Amount per 627 g
1 serving (22.1 oz)

Calories 875
From fat 711

	Amount	% Daily Value*	Amount	% Daily Value*
	Total Fat 80.9g	124%	Total Carbohydrates 20g	7%
	Saturated 52.4g	262%	Dietary Fiber 4g	16%
	Trans Fat 0.9g		Sugars 13g	
	Cholesterol 284mg	95%	Protein 23g	46%
	Sodium 2005mg	84%		
	Calcium 66% • Iron 10%		Vitamin A 59% • Vitamin C 134%	

* Percent Daily Values are based on 2000 calorie diet. Your Daily Values may be higher or lower depending on your calorie needs.

INSTRUCTIONS:

1. In a large saucepan, melt the butter over medium heat.
2. Add the chopped white onion. Cook for 5 to 6 minutes, or until the mushroom has turned light brown. Set aside.

3. To the same saucepan, add the white onion and cauliflower. Cook for 5 to 6 minutes or until the cauliflower has become tender.
4. Add the heavy cream and vegetable broth. Allow to boil and simmer for 10 minutes.
5. Transfer the contents of the saucepan into a blender. Blend until smooth.
6. Transfer the soup to a serving bowl. Top with feta cheese and chives. Serve while hot.

Cream Cheese Scrambled Eggs

INGREDIENTS	Protein	Fat	Carbs
2 eggs	11.05 g	8.37 g	0.63 g
1/2 cup cream cheese	6.88 g	39.72 g	4.72 g
1/4 cup heavy cream	0.62 g	11.1 g	0.84 g
1/4 tbsp thyme	0.03 g	0.01 g	0.15 g
1 tsp oregano	0.16 g	0.08 g	1.24 g
1 tbsp butter	0.12 g	11.52 g	0.01 g

Nutrition Facts

Amount per 251 g
1 serving (8.8 oz)

Calories 733
From fat 624

Amount	% Daily Value*	Amount	% Daily Value*
Total Fat 70.8g	109%	Total Carbohydrates 8g	3%
Saturated 39.4g	197%	Dietary Fiber 1g	3%
Trans Fat 0.5g		Sugars 5g	
Cholesterol 527mg	176%	Protein 19g	38%
Sodium 652mg	27%		
Calcium 22% • Iron 15%		Vitamin A 58% • Vitamin C 2%	

* Percent Daily Values are based on 2000 calorie diet. Your Daily Values may be higher or lower depending on your calorie needs.

INSTRUCTIONS:

1. In a large bowl, combine the eggs, cream cheese, heavy cream, thyme, and oregano. Whisk together until well-combined.

2. Melt the butter in a frying pan over low heat.
3. Pour the egg mixture into the frying pan and cook for 3 to 4 minutes. Make sure to stir the eggs occasionally to keep them soft and creamy.
4. Season with salt and pepper, if desired.
5. Serve immediately.

Mediterranean Zoodles

INGREDIENTS	Protein	Fat	Carbs
1 zucchini	2.37 g	0.63 g	6.1 g
2 tbsp olive oil	0 g	27 g	0 g
1 cup spinach	0.86 g	0.12 g	1.09 g
1 tbsp butter	0.12 g	11.52 g	0.01 g
1 tbsp garlic, chopped	0.54 g	0.04 g	2.81 g
1 tbsp parsley	0.11 g	0.03 g	0.24 g
1/2 tbsp olives, sliced	0.04 g	0.45 g	0.26 g
1/2 cup feta cheese, crumbled	10.66 g	15.96 g	3.07 g
1/4 cup walnuts, chopped	7.53 g	18.57 g	3 g

Nutrition Facts

Amount per 390 g
1 serving (13.8 oz)

Calories 791
From fat 646

	Amount	% Daily Value*	Amount	% Daily Value*
Total Fat 74.3g		114%	Total Carbohydrates 17g	6%
Saturated 23.6g		118%	Dietary Fiber 5g	21%
Trans Fat 0.5g			Sugars 9g	
Cholesterol 97mg		32%	Protein 22g	44%
Sodium 854mg		36%		
Calcium 48% • Iron 20%			Vitamin A 85% • Vitamin C 86%	

* Percent Daily Values are based on 2000 calorie diet. Your Daily Values may be higher or lower depending on your calorie needs.

INSTRUCTIONS:
1. Using a spiralizer, cut the zucchini into thin strips.

2. Press the sliced zucchini between kitchen towels and squeeze out as much moisture as possible. Repeat this process two more times. Set aside.
3. In a large frying pan, melt the butter over low heat. Add the olive oil.
4. Add the chopped garlic and cook until fragrant, about 2 to 3 minutes.
5. Add the spinach and cook just until wilted, which should only take 1 to 2 minutes.
6. Add the olives and stir well.
7. Add the zoodles into the frying pan and stir well, making sure that each strand is covered by the sauce.
8. Add the parsley. Mix well.
9. Transfer the zoodles to a serving bowl. Top with walnuts and feta cheese right before serving.

Roasted Tofu and Asparagus

INGREDIENTS	Protein	Fat	Carbs
4 spears asparagus	0.31 g	0.02 g	0.54 g
1 cup firm tofu, diced	39.77 g	21.97 g	10.76 g
1/2 tbsp garlic, chopped	0.27 g	0.02 g	1.42 g
1/2 tbsp sesame oil	0 g	6.8 g	0 g
1/2 tbsp soy sauce	0.64 g	0.02 g	0.4 g
1/2 tbsp sesame seeds	0.82 g	2.45 g	0.47 g
1 tbsp cilantro, chopped	0.02 g	0.01 g	0.04 g
1/2 tbsp chives, chopped	0.05 g	0.01 g	0.07 g
1 tbsp olive oil	0 g	13.5 g	0 g

<table>
<tr><td rowspan="2">Nutrition Facts

Amount per 304 g
1 serving (10.7 oz)

Calories 584
  From fat 385</td><td>Amount</td><td>% Daily Value*</td><td>Amount</td><td>% Daily Value*</td></tr>
<tr><td colspan="4">
<table>
<tr><td>Total Fat 44.8g</td><td>69%</td><td>Total Carbohydrates 14g</td><td>5%</td></tr>
<tr><td>Saturated 6.4g</td><td>32%</td><td>Dietary Fiber 7g</td><td>27%</td></tr>
<tr><td>Trans Fat 0g</td><td></td><td>Sugars 0g</td><td></td></tr>
<tr><td>Cholesterol 0mg</td><td>0%</td><td>Protein 42g</td><td>84%</td></tr>
<tr><td>Sodium 294mg</td><td>12%</td><td></td><td></td></tr>
<tr><td>Calcium 174% · Iron 42%</td><td></td><td>Vitamin A 13% · Vitamin C 6%</td><td></td></tr>
</table>
* Percent Daily Values are based on 2000 calorie diet. Your Daily Values may be higher or lower depending on your calorie needs.
</td></tr>
</table>

INSTRUCTIONS:

1. Preheat the oven to 400 F.
2. Line a baking tray with parchment paper.
3. Place the asparagus and diced tofu on the baking tray
4. Add the garlic, sesame oil, olive oil, soy sauce, and sesame seeds. Toss all ingredients together until the asparagus and tofu have are well-coated.
5. Bake in the oven for 25 to 30 minutes, or until the asparagus has turned bright green.
6. Remove from the oven and transfer to a serving bowl.
7. Sprinkle with the chopped cilantro and chives before serving.

Keto Fried Mac and Cheese

INGREDIENTS	Protein	Fat	Carbs
1 1/2 cups cauliflower, chopped	3.08 g	0.45 g	7.98 g
3/4 cup cheddar, shredded	20.39 g	28.68 g	1.13 g
2 eggs	11.05 g	8.37 g	0.63 g
1 tsp paprika	0.33 g	0.3 g	1.24 g
1 tsp turmeric	0.29 g	0.1 g	2.01 g
1 1/2 tbsp olive oil	0 g	20.3 g	0 g

<table>
<tr><td rowspan="2">Nutrition Facts

Amount per 359 g
1 serving (12.7 oz)

Calories 706
From fat 520</td><td colspan="2">Amount</td><td>% Daily Value*</td><td colspan="2">Amount</td><td>% Daily Value*</td></tr>
</table>

Amount	% Daily Value*	Amount	% Daily Value*
Total Fat 58.2g	90%	**Total Carbohydrates** 13g	4%
Saturated 22.3g	111%	Dietary Fiber 5g	19%
Trans Fat 1g		Sugars 4g	
Cholesterol 414mg	138%	**Protein** 35g	70%
Sodium 722mg	30%		
Calcium 67% • **Iron** 26%		**Vitamin A** 49% • **Vitamin C** 129%	

Amount per 359 g, 1 serving (12.7 oz). Calories 706, From fat 520.

* Percent Daily Values are based on 2000 calorie diet. Your Daily Values may be higher or lower depending on your calorie needs.

INSTRUCTIONS:

1. Cook the chopped cauliflower in a steamer for 10 minutes, or until tender.
2. Wrap the cooked cauliflower with a kitchen towel and squeeze out as much moisture as possible. Repeat this process two more times.
3. In a large bowl, combine the ground cauliflower, shredded cheddar cheese, eggs, paprika, and turmeric. Mix well until all ingredients are well-incorporated.
4. Separate the mash into equal portions and form patties that are approximately half an inch thick.
5. Preheat the olive oil in a frying pan over high heat.
6. Fry the patties, making sure that the frying pan does not get crowded. Cook each patty for 3 to 4 minutes on each side, or until golden brown.
7. Set aside and allow to cool for 10 minutes before serving.

Pesto Mug Cake

INGREDIENTS	Protein	Fat	Carbs
1 egg	5.53 g	4.18 g	0.32 g
2 tbsp butter	0.24 g	23.04 g	0.02 g

3 tbsp almond flour	5.08 g	11.98 g	5.17 g
1/2 tsp baking powder	0 g	0.01 g	1.17 g
1 1/2 tbsp pesto sauce	2.35 g	13.2 g	0.96 g
1/2 tbsp salsa	0.14 g	0.02 g	0.6 g
1/2 tbsp cheddar, shredded	1.92 g	2.71 g	0.11 g

Nutrition Facts

Amount per 138 g
1 serving (4.9 oz)

Calories 571
From fat 480

	Amount	% Daily Value*	Amount	% Daily Value*
Total Fat	55.1g	85%	Total Carbohydrates 8g	3%
Saturated	20.7g	103%	Dietary Fiber 3g	14%
Trans Fat	1g		Sugars 2g	
Cholesterol	237mg	79%	Protein 15g	31%
Sodium	579mg	24%		
Calcium 32% • Iron 13%			Vitamin A 27% • Vitamin C 2%	

* Percent Daily Values are based on 2000 calorie diet. Your Daily Values may be higher or lower depending on your calorie needs.

INSTRUCTIONS:

1. In a large mug, combine the egg, almond flour, butter, baking powder, and pesto sauce. Add a pinch of salt. Whisk together until well-combined.
2. Microwave the mug on high for 75 seconds.
3. Remove the mug from the microwave and turn over on a plate. Lightly tap the bottom and the sides of the mug to dislodge the cake.
4. Top the pesto cake with salsa and shredded cheddar. Serve while hot.

Cheesy Cauliflower Grits

INGREDIENTS	Protein	Fat	Carbs
2 cups cauliflower, chopped	4.11 g	0.6 g	10.64 g
1/2 cup heavy cream	1.23 g	22.2 g	1.67 g
1/2 cup cheddar	15.87 g	22.32 g	0.88 g

1 tbsp butter	0.12 g	11.52 g	0.01 g
1 tsp paprika	0.33 g	0.3 g	1.24 g
1 tbsp olive oil	0 g	13.5 g	0 g
1 cup white mushrooms, sliced	2.97 g	0.33 g	3.13 g

Nutrition Facts

Amount per 1 serving (16.4 oz)

Calories 777
From fat 627

Amount	% Daily Value*	Amount	% Daily Value*
Total Fat 70.8g	109%	Total Carbohydrates 18g	6%
Saturated 36.1g	181%	Dietary Fiber 6g	24%
Trans Fat 1.3g		Sugars 8g	
Cholesterol 180mg	60%	Protein 25g	49%
Sodium 610mg	25%		
Calcium 54% • Iron 12%		Vitamin A 61% • Vitamin C 176%	

* Percent Daily Values are based on 2000 calorie diet. Your Daily Values may be higher or lower depending on your calorie needs.

INSTRUCTIONS:

1. Place the chopped cauliflower inside a food processor. Pulse until you get a fine to very fine texture.
2. Place the olive oil inside a large saucepan over medium heat.
3. Add the white mushrooms. Cook while stirring for about 7 to 8 minutes, or until the mushrooms have turned a light brown. Set aside.
4. To the same saucepan, add the butter.
5. Add the ground cauliflower and stir. Cook for 4 to 5 minutes.
6. Add the heavy cream and stir well. Allow to boil and simmer for 10 minutes.
7. Add the cheddar and paprika. Stir well.
8. Ladle the grits to a serving bowl and top with the cooked mushroom. Serve while hot.

Sesame and Almond Asian Zoodles

INGREDIENTS	Protein	Fat	Carbs
1 zucchini	1.43 g	0.38 g	3.67 g
1/2 cup firm tofu, diced	19.88 g	10.99 g	5.38 g
1/2 cup broccoli, chopped	0.63 g	0.1 g	0.57 g
1/2 tbsp sesame oil	0 g	6.8 g	0 g
2 tbsp soy sauce	2.57 g	0.09 g	1.59 g
2 tbsp sesame oil	0 g	27.2 g	0 g
1/2 tbsp garlic, chopped	0.27 g	0.02 g	1.42 g
1 tbsp almond butter	3.35 g	8.88 g	3.01 g
1/2 tbsp sesame seeds	0.82 g	2.45 g	0.47 g

Nutrition Facts

Amount per 351 g
1 serving (12.4 oz)

Calories 654
From fat 492

	Amount	% Daily Value*	Amount	% Daily Value*
Total Fat	56.9g	88%	Total Carbohydrates 16g	5%
Saturated	7.6g	38%	Dietary Fiber 7g	28%
Trans Fat	0g		Sugars 4g	
Cholesterol	0mg	0%	Protein 29g	58%
Sodium	1059mg	44%		
Calcium	98%	Iron 31%	Vitamin A 19%	Vitamin C 45%

* Percent Daily Values are based on 2000 calorie diet. Your Daily Values may be higher or lower depending on your calorie needs.

INSTRUCTIONS:

1. Preheat the oven to 400 F.
2. Prepare a baking tray by lining it with parchment paper.
3. Combine the tofu, broccoli, 1/2 tbsp of sesame oil, and garlic on the baking tray. Toss around to combine all the ingredients.
4. Baking in the oven for 20 to 25 minutes, or until the tofu has become firm and the broccoli has become bright green.
5. Remove the baking tray from the oven and set aside.
6. Using a spiralizer, cut the zucchini into thin strands.

7. Squeeze excess moisture out of the zucchini using clean kitchen towels. Repeat this step two more times.
8. In a large bowl, combine the zoodles with the cooked broccoli and tofu.
9. In a smaller bowl, combine the soy sauce, 2 tbsp sesame oil, almond butter, and sesame seeds. Whisk together.
10. Place the sauce in a saucepan and allow to simmer under low heat.
11. Toss in the zoodles and continue cooking for 2 to 3 minutes, or until the zoodles have started to become tender.
12. Serve while hot.

Vegetable and Tofu Curry

INGREDIENTS	Protein	Fat	Carbs
1/2 cup broccoli, chopped	1.28 g	0.17 g	3.02 g
1 cup spinach	0.86 g	0.12 g	1.09 g
1/4 cup eggplant, diced	0.2 g	0.04 g	1.21 g
1/2 cup red onion, sliced	0.06 g	0.01 g	0.47 g
1/2 tbsp ginger	0.05 g	0.02 g	0.53 g
1.2 tbsp garlic	0.27 g	0.02 g	1.42 g
2 tsp fish sauce	0.61 g	0 g	0.44 g
2 tsp soy sauce	0.76 g	1.92 g	2.64 g
1/2 cup coconut milk	2.28 g	24.1 g	3.18 g
1/2 tbsp curry powder	0.46 g	0.45 g	1.79 g
1/2 cup firm tofu	19.88 g	10.99 g	5.38 g
1/2 cup vegetable broth	0 g	0 g	1.5 g
2 tbsp olive oil	0 g	27	0 g

<table>
<tr><td rowspan="6">Nutrition Facts

Amount per 519 g
1 serving (18.3 oz)

Calories 734
From fat 557</td><td>Amount</td><td>% Daily Value*</td><td>Amount</td><td>% Daily Value*</td></tr>
<tr><td>Total Fat 64.8g</td><td>100%</td><td>Total Carbohydrates 23g</td><td>8%</td></tr>
<tr><td>Saturated 27.1g</td><td>136%</td><td>Dietary Fiber 8g</td><td>30%</td></tr>
<tr><td>Trans Fat 0g</td><td></td><td>Sugars 6g</td><td></td></tr>
<tr><td>Cholesterol 0mg</td><td>0%</td><td>Protein 27g</td><td>53%</td></tr>
<tr><td>Sodium 1648mg</td><td>69%</td><td></td><td></td></tr>
<tr><td colspan="3">Calcium 97% • Iron 52%</td><td colspan="2">Vitamin A 71% • Vitamin C 88%</td></tr>
<tr><td colspan="5">* Percent Daily Values are based on 2000 calorie diet. Your Daily Values may be higher or lower depending on your calorie needs.</td></tr>
</table>

INSTRUCTIONS:

1. In a large saucepan, heat the olive oil over medium heat.
2. Add the garlic, red onion, and ginger. Cook for 2 to 3 minutes until fragrant.
3. Add the broccoli and eggplant. Stir while cooking for 5 to 6 minutes or until tender.
4. Add the coconut milk, vegetable broth, fish sauce, soy sauce, and curry powder. Stir well and bring to a boil.
5. Add the tofu. Simmer for 10 minutes.
6. Add the spinach. Cook for an additional 2 minutes.
7. Ladle the curry into a bowl and serve while hot.

Cheesy Keto Waffles

INGREDIENTS	Protein	Fat	Carbs
2 cups cauliflower, chopped	4.11 g	0.6 g	10.64 g
2 eggs	11.05 g	8.37 g	0.63 g
1 cup collard greens	1.09 g	0.22 g	1.95 g
1 tbsp thyme	0.13 g	0.04 g	0.59 g
1 tbsp green onion, chopped	0.06 g	0.03 g	0.34 g
1 tsp garlic powder	0.51 g	0.02 g	2.25 g
1/4 cup cheddar, shredded	6.8 g	9.57 g	0.38 g

| 1/4 cup mozzarella, shredded | 8.97 g | 0 g | 0.99 g |
| 2 tbsp butter | 0.24 g | 23.04 g | 0.02 g |

<table>
<tr><td colspan="2">Nutrition Facts</td><td>Amount</td><td>% Daily Value*</td><td>Amount</td><td>% Daily Value*</td></tr>
<tr><td colspan="2" rowspan="6">Amount per 435 g
1 serving (15.3 oz)

Calories 564
From fat 372</td><td>Total Fat 41.9g</td><td>64%</td><td>Total Carbohydrates 18g</td><td>6%</td></tr>
<tr><td>Saturated 23.1g</td><td>116%</td><td>Dietary Fiber 7g</td><td>28%</td></tr>
<tr><td>Trans Fat 1.3g</td><td></td><td>Sugars 5g</td><td></td></tr>
<tr><td>Cholesterol 422mg</td><td>141%</td><td>Protein 33g</td><td>66%</td></tr>
<tr><td>Sodium 773mg</td><td>32%</td><td></td><td></td></tr>
<tr><td colspan="2">Calcium 67% • Iron 19%</td><td>Vitamin A 75% • Vitamin C 201%</td><td></td></tr>
<tr><td colspan="6">* Percent Daily Values are based on 2000 calorie diet. Your Daily Values may be higher or lower depending on your calorie needs.</td></tr>
</table>

INSTRUCTIONS:

1. In a food processor, combine the cauliflower, collard greens, thyme, and green onion. Pulse until you get a very fine texture.
2. Transfer the contents of the food processor into a large mixing bowl.
3. Add the eggs, butter, garlic powder, cheddar, and mozzarella to the mixing bowl. Stir well until a batter is formed.
4. Heat your waffle iron according to instructions. Scoop the batter into the waffle iron, making sure that it is evenly distributed.
5. Cook the waffle according to the instructions in your waffle iron.
6. Remove from the waffle iron and serve while hot.

Spicy Roasted Tofu in Soft Tacos

INGREDIENTS	Protein	Fat	Carbs
1/2 cup firm tofu	19.88 g	10.99 g	5.38 g
1 tbsp sesame oil	0 g	13.6 g	0 g
1 tsp paprika	0.33 g	0.3 g	1.24 g
1/2 tbsp garlic	0.27 g	0.02 g	1.42 g
1/2 tbsp sesame seeds	0.82 g	2.45 g	0.47 g
1 cup romaine lettuce, shredded	0.58 g	0.14 g	1.55 g
1 tbsp red onion, chopped	0.11 g	0.01 g	0.93 g
1 egg	5.53 g	4.18 g	0.32 g
1/2 cup almond flour	10.05 g	23.72 g	10.24 g
1 tbsp olive oil	0 g	13.5 g	0 g

Nutrition Facts

Amount per 312 g
1 serving (11 oz)

Calories 810
From fat 592

	Amount	% Daily Value*	Amount	% Daily Value*
	Total Fat 68.9g	106%	Total Carbohydrates 22g	7%
	Saturated 9g	45%	Dietary Fiber 11g	45%
	Trans Fat 0g		Sugars 4g	
	Cholesterol 164mg	55%	Protein 38g	75%
	Sodium 89mg	4%		
	Calcium 105% • Iron 40%		Vitamin A 114% • Vitamin C	7%

* Percent Daily Values are based on 2000 calorie diet. Your Daily Values may be higher or lower depending on your calorie needs.

INSTRUCTIONS:

1. Preheat the oven to 400 F.
2. Prepare a baking tray by lining it with parchment paper.
3. In the baking tray, combine the tofu, sesame oil, paprika, garlic, and sesame seeds. Toss together until all the tofu has been coated.
4. Bake in the oven for 25 to 30 minutes, or until the tofu has become firm.
5. Remove from the oven and set aside to cool.

6. In a small mixing bowl, combine the egg, almond, flour, and olive oil. Whisk together until you get a smooth batter.
7. Heat a frying pan over low heat.
8. Cook the tacos one at a time by scooping the batter to the frying pan and cooking for half a minute on each side. Repeat this step until all the batter has been consumed.
9. Toss the cooked tofu with the shredded lettuce and red onion.
10. Spoon the tofu mixture into each taco shell.
11. Serve immediately.

High-Protein Granola Bark

INGREDIENTS	Protein	Fat	Carbs
1 1/2 tbsp desiccated coconut	1.27 g	16.58 g	5.16 g
1 1/2 tbsp sunflower seeds	2.72 g	6.74 g	2.62 g
1 1/2 tbsp pumpkin seeds	3.31 g	5.44 g	1.63 g
1 tbsp poppy seeds	1.58 g	3.66 g	2.48 g
1 1/2 tbsp walnuts, chopped	2.82 g	6.94 g	1.12 g
1/4 cup coconut oil	0 g	54.5 g	0 g
1/2 tsp cinnamon powder	0.05 g	0.02 g	1.05 g
1 tbsp protein powder	5.03 g	1.89 g	2.04 g

<table>
<tr><td rowspan="6">Nutrition Facts
Amount per   136 g
1 serving (4.8 oz)

Calories   941
  From fat 816</td><td>Amount</td><td>% Daily Value*</td><td>Amount</td><td>% Daily Value*</td></tr>
<tr><td>Total Fat 95.8g</td><td>147%</td><td>Total Carbohydrates 16g</td><td>5%</td></tr>
<tr><td>Saturated 64.4g</td><td>322%</td><td>Dietary Fiber 6g</td><td>23%</td></tr>
<tr><td>Trans Fat 0.1g</td><td></td><td>Sugars 2g</td><td></td></tr>
<tr><td>Cholesterol 2mg</td><td>1%</td><td>Protein 17g</td><td>34%</td></tr>
<tr><td>Sodium 77mg</td><td>3%</td><td></td><td></td></tr>
</table>

Calcium 22% • **Iron** 26%   **Vitamin A** 6% • **Vitamin C** 7%

* Percent Daily Values are based on 2000 calorie diet. Your Daily Values may be higher or lower depending on your calorie needs.

INSTRUCTIONS:

1. Preheat the oven to 350 F.
2. Line a large baking tray with parchment paper.
3. Into the baking tray, toss together the desiccated coconut, sunflower seeds, pumpkin seeds, poppy seeds, protein powder, and chopped walnuts.
4. Melt the coconut oil in a small frying pan over low heat. Stir in the cinnamon powder.
5. Pour the melted coconut oil over the granola mix. Stir thoroughly until everything has been coated with the coconut oil.
6. Bake in the oven for 15 to 20 minutes, or until the granola bark has started to become firm.
7. Allow the granola bark to cool and further harden. It is best served in room temperature.

Basic Mushroom Omelet

INGREDIENTS	Protein	Fat	Carbs
1 cup white mushrooms, sliced	2.16 g	0.24 g	2.28 g
1 tbsp olive oil	0 g	13.5 g	0 g
2 eggs	11.05 g	8.37 g	0.63 g
2 tbsp heavy cream	0.62 g	11.1 g	0.84 g

1 tbsp butter	0.12 g	11.52 g	0.01 g
1/2 cup cheddar, shredded	13.58 g	19.11 g	0.75 g
1 tsp oregano, ground	0.16 g	0.08 g	1.24 g

Nutrition Facts

Amount per 274 g
1 serving (9.7 oz)

Calories 700
From fat 568

	Amount	% Daily Value*	Amount	% Daily Value*
Total Fat 63.9g		98%	**Total Carbohydrates** 6g	2%
Saturated 29.8g		149%	Dietary Fiber 2g	6%
Trans Fat 1.2g			Sugars 3g	
Cholesterol 457mg		152%	**Protein** 28g	55%
Sodium 596mg		25%		
Calcium 49% • **Iron** 15%			**Vitamin A** 37% • **Vitamin C** 3%	

* Percent Daily Values are based on 2000 calorie diet. Your Daily Values may be higher or lower depending on your calorie needs.

INSTRUCTIONS:

1. Heat the olive oil in a frying pan over high heat.
2. Toss in the white mushrooms and cook while stirring. Cook for 8 to 9 minutes, or until the mushrooms have turned light brown.
3. Remove from the heat and set aside.
4. In a medium-sized mixing bowl, whisk together the eggs and heavy cream.
5. Melt the butter in the frying pan over medium heat.
6. Pour in the egg mixture.
7. When the bottom of the omelet has started to become firm (after about 2 minutes), pour in the cooked mushroom and shredded cheddar over the top.
8. Continue cooking for one more minute before turning off the heat.
9. Fold the omelet inwards and transfer to a serving plate.
10. Sprinkle oregano over the top of the omelet before serving.

Fried Zucchini Patties with Pesto Sauce

INGREDIENTS	Protein	Fat	Carbs
1 medium zucchini	2.37 g	0.63 g	6.1 g
1 egg	5.53 g	4.18 g	0.32 g
1/4 cup almond flour	5.03 g	11.88 g	5.13 g
1/2 tsp garlic powder	0.26 g	0.01 g	1.16 g
1/2 tsp cumin	0.2 g	0.24 g	0.49 g
1 tbsp butter	0.12 g	11.52 g	0.01 g
2 tbsp olive oil	0 g	27 g	0 g
1 tbsp pesto sauce	1.56 g	8.8 g	0.64 g
1/2 cup soft tofu, cubes	8.12 g	4.58 g	2.23 g
1 tbsp sesame seeds	1.64 g	4.9 g	0.94 g

Nutrition Facts

Amount per 455 g
1 serving (16 oz)

Calories 796
From fat 641

	Amount	% Daily Value*	Amount	% Daily Value*
Total Fat 73.7g		113%	Total Carbohydrates 17g	6%
Saturated 16.4g		82%	Dietary Fiber 7g	26%
Trans Fat 0.5g			Sugars 7g	
Cholesterol 197mg		66%	Protein 25g	50%
Sodium 331mg		14%		
Calcium 32% • Iron 31%			Vitamin A 24% • Vitamin C 60%	

* Percent Daily Values are based on 2000 calorie diet. Your Daily Values may be higher or lower depending on your calorie needs.

INSTRUCTIONS:

1. Cut the zucchini into very small and thin strips using a mandolin slicer. If you don't have a mandolin slicer, a knife will do.

2. In a large mixing bowl, combine the sliced zucchini, egg, almond flour, soft tofu, sesame seeds, garlic powder, and cumin. Stir thoroughly until all ingredients are well-combined.

3. Melt the butter with olive oil in a frying pan over medium heat.

4. Scoop the batter into the frying pan and flatten into a patty. Cook on each side until it has turned golden brown, about 4 to 5 minutes.
5. Repeat the previous step until all the batter has been cooked.
6. Allow the patties to cool for ten minutes.
7. Scoop pesto sauce over the top of each patty before serving.

Stuffed Portobello Pizzas

INGREDIENTS	Protein	Fat	Carbs
3 pieces portobello, whole	5.32 g	0.88 g	9.75 g
1 cup cheddar, shredded	27.17 g	38.22 g	1.5 g
3 tbsp ready-to-serve salsa	0.83 g	0.09 g	3.63 g
1/2 cup spinach, chopped	0.43 g	0.06 g	0.54 g
1/2 cup sweet red pepper, diced	0.46 g	0.14 g	2.77 g
1/2 tbsp olives, sliced	0.04 g	0.45 g	0.26 g
1 tbsp olive oil	0 g	13.5 g	0 g

Nutrition Facts

Amount per 498 g
1 serving (17.6 oz)

Calories 672
From fat 477

	Amount	% Daily Value*		Amount	% Daily Value*
Total Fat	53.3g	82%	Total Carbohydrates	18g	6%
Saturated	24g	120%	Dietary Fiber	6g	23%
Trans Fat	1.3g		Sugars	11g	
Cholesterol	115mg	38%	Protein	34g	68%
Sodium	1176mg	49%			
Calcium	81% • Iron 11%		Vitamin A	85% • Vitamin C 107%	

* Percent Daily Values are based on 2000 calorie diet. Your Daily Values may be higher or lower depending on your calorie needs.

INSTRUCTIONS:

1. Preheat the oven to 450 F.
2. Remove the stems from the portobello mushrooms. Wash them thoroughly and pat them dry.
3. Place the mushrooms on a baking try, cap side down.
4. Scoop salsa into each mushroom and spread evenly.
5. Sprinkle cheddar over each mushroom. Top with spinach, sweet peppers, and olives.
6. Drizzle olive oil over the top of each mushroom.
7. Place the baking tray in the oven and cook for 25 to 30 minutes, or until the mushroom has become soft.
8. Remove the tray from the oven. Allow to cool for 10 minutes before serving.

Cheesy Roasted Broccoli and Cauliflower

INGREDIENTS	Protein	Fat	Carbs
3 cups broccoli, chopped	3.8 g	0.59 g	3.42 g
1/2 cup cheddar, shredded	15.87 g	22.32 g	0.88 g
1 tbsp garlic, chopped	0.54 g	0.04 g	2.81 g
2 tbsp olive oil	0 g	27 g	0 g
1 tsp oregano	0.09 g	0.04 g	0.69 g
1 cup cauliflower, chopped	2.05 g	0.3 g	5.32 g

Nutrition Facts	Amount	% Daily Value*	Amount	% Daily Value*
Amount per 330 g 1 serving (11.6 oz)	**Total Fat** 50.3g	77%	**Total Carbohydrates** 13g	4%
	Saturated 16.7g	84%	Dietary Fiber 6g	24%
	Trans Fat 0.8g		Sugars 3g	
Calories 575	**Cholesterol** 67mg	22%	**Protein** 22g	45%
From fat 448	**Sodium** 499mg	21%		
	Calcium 63% • **Iron** 21%		**Vitamin A** 76% • **Vitamin C** 131%	

* Percent Daily Values are based on 2000 calorie diet. Your Daily Values may be higher or lower depending on your calorie needs.

INSTRUCTIONS:

1. Preheat the oven to 350 F.
2. Place the olive oil in a small mixing bowl and toss in the chopped garlic and oregano. Whisk together.
3. In a baking tray, toss the chopped cauliflower and broccoli with the olive oil mixture. Make sure that the vegetables are well-coated. Spread them evenly over the baking tray.
4. Sprinkle shredded cheddar over the top of the vegetables.
5. Place the baking tray in the oven and bake for 12 to 15 minutes, or until the vegetables have changed color.
6. Remove from the tray and transfer to a serving dish. Serve immediately.

Two-Cheese Asparagus Frittata

INGREDIENTS	Protein	Fat	Carbs
1/4 cup cheddar, shredded	6.8 g	9.57 g	0.38 g
2 eggs	11.05 g	8.37 g	0.63 g
2 tbsp soft goat cheese	5.93 g	6.75 g	0 g
1 1/2 tbsp butter	0.18 g	17.28 g	0.01 g
4 asparagus spears	1.41 g	0.08 g	2.48 g
1 cup milk	7.69 g	7.98 g	11.66 g

Nutrition Facts	Amount	% Daily Value*	Amount	% Daily Value*
Amount per 478 g 1 serving (16.8 oz)	**Total Fat** 50g	77%	**Total Carbohydrates** 15g	5%
	Saturated 28.4g	142%	Dietary Fiber 1g	5%
	Trans Fat 1.1g		Sugars 14g	
Calories 640 From fat 445	**Cholesterol** 441mg	147%	**Protein** 33g	66%
	Sodium 697mg	29%		
	Calcium 58% • **Iron** 20%		**Vitamin A** 50% • **Vitamin C** 6%	

* Percent Daily Values are based on 2000 calorie diet. Your Daily Values may be higher or lower depending on your calorie needs.

INSTRUCTIONS:

1. Cut the asparagus spears into 1-inch long segments.
2. Melt a pat of butter in a frying pan over medium heat.
3. Cook the asparagus spears in the frying pan for 5 to 6 minutes, or just until they have turned bright green.
4. Remove from the heat and set aside.
5. In a large mixing bowl, whisk together the eggs and milk. Season with salt and pepper if desired.
6. Melt the rest of the butter in the frying pan over low heat.
7. Pour in the egg mixture. Cook for 3 to 4 minutes.
8. Add the goat cheese, cheddar, and cooked asparagus into the frittata. Cook for an additional 2 minutes.
9. Remove from the heat. Transfer the frittata to a plate and serve.

Zoodles Pad Thai

INGREDIENTS	Protein	Fat	Carbs
1 cup firm tofu, diced	39.77 g	21.97 g	10.76 g
1/2 tbsp sesame oil	0 g	6.8 g	0 g
1/2 tbsp sesame seeds	1.64 g	4.9 g	0.94 g
1 medium zucchini	2.37 g	0.63 g	6.1 g

1 tbsp red onion, chopped	0.11 g	0.01 g	0.93 g
1/2 tbsp garlic, chopped	0.27 g	0.02 g	1.42 g
1/2 tbsp ginger, grated	0.05 g	0.02 g	0.53 g
1 tbsp fish sauce	0.91 g	0 g	0.66 g
1 tbsp lemon juice	0.05 g	0.04 g	1.06 g
1/2 tbsp chili powder	0.54 g	0.57 g	1.99 g
1 tbsp cilantro, chopped	0.02 g	0.01 g	0.04 g
1 tbsp peanuts, ground	3.93 g	8.04 g	3.24 g

Nutrition Facts

Amount per 534 g
1 serving (18.9 oz)

Calories 637
From fat 368

	Amount	% Daily Value*	Amount	% Daily Value*
Total Fat 43g		66%	Total Carbohydrates 28g	9%
Saturated 6.3g		32%	Dietary Fiber 12g	47%
Trans Fat 0g			Sugars 7g	
Cholesterol 0mg		0%	Protein 50g	99%
Sodium 1680mg		70%		
Calcium 180% • Iron 51%			Vitamin A 41% • Vitamin C 74%	

* Percent Daily Values are based on 2000 calorie diet. Your Daily Values may be higher or lower depending on your calorie needs.

INSTRUCTIONS:

1. Preheat the oven to 400 F.
2. Cut the zucchini into zoodles using a spiralizer.
3. Squeeze out excess moisture from by pressing between clean kitchen towels. Repeat this step two more times. Set the zoodles aside.
4. In a baking tray, toss together the cubes of firm tofu, sesame oil, and sesame seeds.
5. Bake the tofu in the oven for 20 to 24 minutes, or until the tofu has turned light brown.
6. Remove from the oven and set aside.
7. In a large saucepan, combine red onion, garlic, ginger, chili powder, fish sauce, and lemon juice. Turn on the heat to medium and allow the mixture to simmer.

8. Add the zoodles and the cooked tofu. Stir while continuing to cook for an additional 3 minutes.
9. Turn off the heat. Transfer the pad thai to a serving plate.
10. Sprinkle with cilantro and peanuts right before serving

.

Cheesy Brussels Sprouts

INGREDIENTS	Protein	Fat	Carbs
1 1/2 cups brussels sprouts, quartered	4.46 g	0.4 g	11.81 g
1 tbsp olive oil	0 g	13.5 g	0 g
1 tbsp butter	0.12 g	11.52 g	0.01 g
1 tbsp white onion, chopped	0.11 g	0.01 g	0.93 g
1/2 cup heavy cream	1.23 g	22.2 g	1.67 g
3 tbsp sour cream	1.26 g	3.82 g	2.56 g
1/4 cup cheddar, shredded	6.8 g	9.57 g	0.38 g
1/4 cup mozzarella, shredded	6.21 g	6.26 g	0.61 g

Nutrition Facts

Amount per 322 g
1 serving (11.4 oz)

Calories 737
From fat 595

	Amount	% Daily Value*	Amount	% Daily Value*
Total Fat	67.3g	103%	Total Carbohydrates 18g	6%
Saturated	34.6g	173%	Dietary Fiber 5g	21%
Trans Fat	0.8g		Sugars 5g	
Cholesterol	176mg	59%	Protein 20g	40%
Sodium	535mg	22%		
Calcium	48% • Iron 12%		Vitamin A 56% • Vitamin C 189%	

* Percent Daily Values are based on 2000 calorie diet. Your Daily Values may be higher or lower depending on your calorie needs.

INSTRUCTIONS:
1. Place the olive oil in a large saucepan over medium heat.

2. Add the brussels sprouts. Cook for 15 to 18 minutes while stirring occasionally.
3. Remove the brussels sprouts from the pan and set aside.
4. Melt the butter over medium heat.
5. Add the white onion. Cook for 4 to 5 minutes or until tender.
6. Add the heavy cream, sour cream, cheddar, and mozzarella. Lower the heat to a simmer and stir continuously until all the cheese has melted.
7. Add in the cooked brussels sprouts. Stir well. Continue cooking for 5 more minutes.
8. Transfer the contents of the saucepan into a serving plate. Allow to cool for 5 minutes before serving.

Quick Caprese Salad

INGREDIENTS	Protein	Fat	Carbs
2 tomatoes	2.16 g	0.49 g	9.57 g
1 cup mozzarella, shredded	35.82 g	0 g	3.96 g
2 tbsp pesto sauce	3.13 g	17.6 g	1.28 g
1/2 tbsp peanuts, ground	3.93 g	8.04 g	3.24 g
2 tbsp olive oil	0 g	27 g	0 g

Nutrition Facts

Amount per 432 g
1 serving (15.2 oz)

Calories 708
From fat 469

	Amount	% Daily Value*	Amount	% Daily Value*
Total Fat	53.1g	82%	Total Carbohydrates 18g	6%
Saturated	7.9g	40%	Dietary Fiber 7g	26%
Trans Fat	0g		Sugars 9g	
Cholesterol	25mg	8%	Protein 45g	90%
Sodium	1237mg	52%		
Calcium 120% • Iron 12%			Vitamin A 59% • Vitamin C 58%	

* Percent Daily Values are based on 2000 calorie diet. Your Daily Values may be higher or lower depending on your calorie needs.

INSTRUCTIONS:

1. Slice the tomatoes into large cubes and place into the serving bowl.
2. Add the mozzarella, pesto sauce, peanuts, and olive oil. Toss well.
3. Serve immediately.

Cheesy Cauliflower Mash

INGREDIENTS	Protein	Fat	Carbs
1 1/2 cups cauliflower, chopped	3.08 g	0.45 g	7.98 g
1/2 cup heavy cream	1.23 g	22.2 g	1.67 g
2 tbsp butter	0.24 g	23.04 g	0.02 g
1 tsp thyme	0.04 g	0.01 g	0.2 g
1 tsp oregano	0.09 g	0.04 g	0.69 g
2 tbsp garlic, chopped	1.08 g	0.09 g	5.62 g
1 tbsp olive oil	0 g	13.5 g	0 g
1 cup mozzarella, shredded	17.91 g	0 g	1.98 g

Nutrition Facts

Amount per 338 g
1 serving (11.9 oz)

Calories 679
From fat 522

Amount	% Daily Value*	Amount	% Daily Value*
Total Fat 59.3g	91%	Total Carbohydrates 18g	6%
Saturated 30.5g	153%	Dietary Fiber 5g	20%
Trans Fat 0.9g		Sugars 6g	
Cholesterol 153mg	51%	Protein 24g	47%
Sodium 677mg	28%		
Calcium 67% • Iron 10%		Vitamin A 38% • Vitamin C 141%	

* Percent Daily Values are based on 2000 calorie diet. Your Daily Values may be higher or lower depending on your calorie needs.

INSTRUCTIONS:

1. In a medium-sized pot, melt the butter with olive oil over medium heat.
2. Add the garlic and cauliflower. Cook while stirring for 8 to 10 minutes, or until the cauliflower has become soft.
3. Add the heavy cream and stir. Lower the heat to a simmer. Continue cooking for 10 minutes.
4. Transfer the contents of the pot to a food processor. Pulse the mixture until the texture hs become smooth.
5. Add the thyme, oregano, and mozzarella to the mash. Pulse again until the additional ingredients have become well-incorporated.
6. Transfer the mash to a bowl and serve immediately.

Simple Roasted Broccoli and Tofu

INGREDIENTS	Protein	Fat	Carbs
1 1/2 cups broccoli, chopped	3.85 g	0.51 g	9.06 g
1 cup firm tofu, diced	39.77 g	21.97 g	10.76 g
1 tbsp sesame oil	0 g	13.6 g	0 g
1 tbsp garlic, chopped	0.54 g	0.04 g	2.81 g
1 tsp paprika	0.33 g	0.3 g	1.24 g
1/2 tbsp sesame seeds	0.82 g	2.45 g	0.47 g
1 tbsp lemon juice	0.05 g	0.04 g	1.06 g
1 tbsp olive oil	0 g	13.5 g	0 g
1/2 tbsp sunflower seeds	0.91 g	2.26 g	0.88 g

<table>
<tr><td rowspan="4">Nutrition Facts

Amount per 450 g
1 serving (15.9 oz)

Calories 725
From fat 470</td><td>Amount</td><td>% Daily Value*</td><td>Amount</td><td>% Daily Value*</td></tr>
</table>

Amount	% Daily Value*	Amount	% Daily Value*
Total Fat 54.7g	84%	**Total Carbohydrates** 26g	9%
Saturated 7.6g	38%	Dietary Fiber 11g	45%
Trans Fat 0g		Sugars 3g	
Cholesterol 0mg	0%	**Protein** 46g	93%
Sodium 86mg	4%		
Calcium 181% • **Iron** 49%		**Vitamin A** 48% • **Vitamin C** 218%	

Nutrition Facts

Amount per 450 g
1 serving (15.9 oz)

Calories 725
From fat 470

* Percent Daily Values are based on 2000 calorie diet. Your Daily Values may be higher or lower depending on your calorie needs.

INSTRUCTIONS:

1. Preheat the oven to 450 F.
2. Line a baking tray with parchment paper.
3. Place the broccoli and firm tofu on the baking tray.
4. Sprinkle the sesame oil, olive oil, garlic, paprika, sesame seeds, and sunflower seeds to the baking tray.
5. Toss the ingredients well, making sure that the tofu and broccoli are well-coated.
6. Bake in the oven for 25 to 28 minutes.
7. Remove the tray from the oven and transfer the contents to a serving bowl.
8. Sprinkle lemon juice right before serving.

High-Protein Coconut and Chocolate Smoothie

INGREDIENTS	Protein	Fat	Carbs
1/2 cup coconut milk	2.28 g	24.1 g	3.18 g
1/4 cup milk	1.92 g	1.99 g	2.92 g
1/2 tbsp cacao powder	0.62 g	3.41 g	3.67 g
3 tbsp protein powder	15.08 g	5.66 g	6.11 g
2 tbsp coconut oil	0 g	27.2 g	0 g

1/4 tsp vanilla extract	0 g	0 g	0.14 g
1/4 tsp cinnamon powder	0.03 g	0.01 g	0.56 g

Nutrition Facts

Amount per 244 g
1 serving (8.6 oz)

Calories 683
From fat 536

	Amount	% Daily Value*	Amount	% Daily Value*
Total Fat 62.4g		96%	**Total Carbohydrates** 17g	6%
Saturated 48.5g		243%	Dietary Fiber 4g	14%
Trans Fat 0.1g			Sugars 7g	
Cholesterol 13mg		4%	**Protein** 20g	40%
Sodium 151mg		6%		
Calcium 27% • **Iron** 42%			**Vitamin A** 19% • **Vitamin C** 19%	

* Percent Daily Values are based on 2000 calorie diet. Your Daily Values may be higher or lower depending on your calorie needs.

INSTRUCTIONS:

1. Combine all ingredients in a blender. Add 4 to 5 ice cubes.
2. Blend until smooth.
3. Serve smoothie immediately, while still chilled.

Keto Vegetarian Lasagna

INGREDIENTS	Protein	Fat	Carbs
1 medium zucchini	2.37 g	0.63 g	6.1 g
1 cup ricotta cheese	27.92 g	32.19 g	7.54 g
1 1/2 tbsp canned tomato sauce	0.37 g	0.09 g	1.62 g
1/2 tbsp oregano	0.72 g	0.34 g	5.51 g
1 tbsp olive oil	0 g	13.5 g	0 g

Nutrition Facts

Amount per 496 g
1 serving (17.5 oz)

Calories 613
From fat 411

	Amount	% Daily Value*	Amount	% Daily Value*
Total Fat 46.8g		72%	**Total Carbohydrates** 21g	7%
Saturated 22.7g		114%	Dietary Fiber 6g	23%
Trans Fat 0g			Sugars 7g	
Cholesterol 126mg		42%	**Protein** 31g	63%
Sodium 371mg		15%		
Calcium 68% • **Iron** 28%			**Vitamin A** 35% • **Vitamin C** 62%	

* Percent Daily Values are based on 2000 calorie diet. Your Daily Values may be higher or lower depending on your calorie needs.

INSTRUCTIONS:

1. Preheat the oven to 400 F.
2. Using a mandolin slicer, slice the zucchini into thin, long strips.
3. Squeeze out excess moisture from the zucchini strips by pressing between kitchen towels. Repeat this process two more times. Set the zucchini strips aside.
4. In a small bowl, mix the tomato sauce, oregano and olive oil.
5. Assemble your lasagna in a small, deep oven-safe dish. Place a layer of tomato sauce mixture on the bottom and top with the zucchini strips, making sure to form a complete layer each time.
6. Top the zucchini layer with another layer of tomato sauce followed by a layer of ricotta cheese.
7. Place another layer of zucchini strips and repeat this process until all ingredients have been used up. Finish up the lasagna with a layer of ricotta cheese on top.
8. Bake the lasagna in the oven for 20 to 25 minutes, or until the top layer has turned golden brown.
9. Remove the lasagna from the oven and allow to cool for about 10 minutes before serving.

Keto-Friendly Pumpkin Soup

INGREDIENTS	Protein	Fat	Carbs
1/2 cup raw pumpkin, cubed	0.58 g	0.06 g	3.77 g
1 cup heavy cream	1.85 g	33.3 g	2.51 g
1 tbsp butter	0.12 g	11.52 g	0.01 g
1 egg	5.53 g	4.18 g	0.32 g
1/2 tsp pumpkin spice	0.05 g	0.11 g	0.62 g

1/2 tsp cinnamon	0.05 g	0.02 g	1.05 g
1/4 tsp vanilla extract	0 g	0 g	0.14 g
2 tbsp ricotta	3.49 g	4.02 g	0.94 g
1 tbsp pumpkin seeds	2.21 g	3.63 g	1.09 g
1/2 cup vegetable broth	0 g	0 g	1.5 g

Nutrition Facts

Amount per 365 g
1 serving (12.9 oz)

Calories 602
From fat 499

Amount	% Daily Value*	Amount	% Daily Value*
Total Fat 56.8g	87%	Total Carbohydrates 12g	4%
Saturated 32.7g	163%	Dietary Fiber 2g	6%
Trans Fat 0.5g		Sugars 6g	
Cholesterol 333mg	111%	Protein 14g	28%
Sodium 704mg	29%		
Calcium 19% • Iron 13%		Vitamin A 145% • Vitamin C 10%	

* Percent Daily Values are based on 2000 calorie diet. Your Daily Values may be higher or lower depending on your calorie needs.

INSTRUCTIONS:

1. In a mixing bowl, whisk together the heavy cream and egg. Set aside.
2. Melt the butter in a large pot over high heat.
3. Add the pumpkin, heavy cream mixture, and vegetable broth to the pot. Heat until boiling.
4. Add the pumpkin spice, cinnamon, and vanilla extract to the pot. Lower the heat to a simmer and cook for an additional 15 to 20 minutes, or until the pumpkin has become tender.
5. Transfer the contents of the bowl to a blender. Blend until smooth.
6. Place the soup on a serving bowl. Add the ricotta cheese while the soup is still hot. Sprinkle pumpkin seeds on top and serve.

Teriyaki Tofu

INGREDIENTS	Protein	Fat	Carbs
1 1/4 cup firm tofu, cubes	49.71 g	27.47 g	13.45 g
1 1/2 tbsp coconut oil	0 g	20.4 g	0 g
1 tbsp sesame oil	0 g	13.6 g	0 g
1/2 tbsp ginger	0.05 g	0.02 g	0.53 g
1 tbsp red onion	0.11 g	0.01 g	0.93 g
2 tbsp soy sauce	2.57 g	0.09 g	1.59 g
1 cup spinach	0.86 g	0.12 g	1.09 g
1/2 tbsp sesame seeds	0.82 g	2.45 g	0.47 g
1/2 tbsp chives, chopped	0.05 g	0.01 g	0.07 g

Nutrition Facts

Amount per 426 g
1 serving (15 oz)

Calories 808
From fat 549

	Amount	% Daily Value*	Amount	% Daily Value*
Total Fat 64.2g		99%	**Total Carbohydrates** 18g	6%
Saturated 24g		120%	Dietary Fiber 9g	35%
Trans Fat 0g			Sugars 1g	
Cholesterol 0mg		0%	**Protein** 54g	108%
Sodium 1092mg		46%		
Calcium 220% • **Iron** 55%			**Vitamin A** 68% • **Vitamin C** 18%	

* Percent Daily Values are based on 2000 calorie diet. Your Daily Values may be higher or lower depending on your calorie needs.

INSTRUCTIONS:

1. Preheat the oven to 400 F.
2. In a baking tray lined with parchment paper, toss together the tofu, sesame oil, and sesame seeds.
3. Bake in the oven for 20 to 25 minutes, or until the tofu has become firm.
4. Remove the tofu from the oven and set aside.
5. In a large frying pan, preheat the coconut oil over medium heat.
6. Add the ginger and red onion to the frying pan. Cook for 2 to 3 minutes, or until fragrant.
7. Add the cooked tofu and soy sauce. Toss together in the pan and cook for an additional 4 to 5 minutes.
8. Add the spinach and allow to wilt for about 2 to 3minutes.

9. Transfer the contents of the pan to a serving dish. Top with chopped chives right before serving.

Ricotta and Cheddar Cheese Fritters

INGREDIENTS	Protein	Fat	Carbs
3/4 cup ricotta cheese	20.94 g	24.14 g	5.65 g
1/2 cup cheddar, shredded	13.58 g	19.11 g	0.75 g
1/2 cup peanut flour	15.66 g	0.17 g	10.41 g
1 egg	5.53 g	4.18 g	0.32 g
1 tsp oregano, ground	0.16 g	0.08 g	1.24 g
2 tbsp olive oil	0 g	27 g	0 g
1 tbsp sour cream	0.42 g	1.27 g	0.85 g
1/2 tbsp lemon juice	0.03 g	0.02 g	0.52 g

Nutrition Facts

Amount per 365 g
1 serving (12.9 oz)

Calories 975
From fat 674

	Amount	% Daily Value*		Amount	% Daily Value*
	Total Fat 76g	117%		**Total Carbohydrates** 20g	7%
	Saturated 32.3g	162%		Dietary Fiber 6g	22%
	Trans Fat 0.7g			Sugars 4g	
	Cholesterol 320mg	107%		**Protein** 56g	113%
	Sodium 648mg	27%			
	Calcium 88% • **Iron** 17%			**Vitamin A** 34% • **Vitamin C** 5%	

* Percent Daily Values are based on 2000 calorie diet. Your Daily Values may be higher or lower depending on your calorie needs.

INSTRUCTIONS:

1. In a large mixing bowl, combine the ricotta cheese, cheddar cheese, egg, peanut flour, and oregano. Mix well until well-combined.
2. Separate the mixture into three equal portions and form them into patties about half an inch thick.
3. Heat the olive oil in a frying pan over medium heat.
4. Fry the cheese fritters one at a time for 2 to 3 minutes on each side.

5. Sprinkle lemon juice over the cooked fritters and place a dollop of sour cream on top of each one before serving.

Spinach and Ricotta Bake

INGREDIENTS	Protein	Fat	Carbs
2 eggs	110.5 g	8.37 g	0.63 g
1/2 cup ricotta	13.96 g	16.1 g	3.77 g
1 cup spinach	0.86 g	0.12 g	1.09 g
1/2 cup heavy cream	1.23 g	22.2 g	1.67 g
1 tbsp garlic, chopped	0.54 g	0.04 g	2.81 g
1/4 tsp nutmeg	0.04 g	0.22 g	0.3 g
1/2 tsp paprika	0.17 g	0.15 g	0.65 g
1 tbsp parsley, chopped	0.11 g	0.03 g	0.24 g
1/4 cup almond flour	5.03 g	11.88 g	5.13 g

Nutrition Facts

Amount per 340 g
1 serving (12 oz)

Calories 714
From fat 516

	Amount	% Daily Value*
Total Fat	59.1g	91%
Saturated	28g	140%
Trans Fat	0g	
Cholesterol	473mg	158%
Sodium	280mg	12%
Calcium 46% • Iron 24%		

	Amount	% Daily Value*
Total Carbohydrates	16g	5%
Dietary Fiber	5g	18%
Sugars	4g	
Protein	33g	66%
Vitamin A 113% • Vitamin C 28%		

* Percent Daily Values are based on 2000 calorie diet. Your Daily Values may be higher or lower depending on your calorie needs.

INSTRUCTIONS:
1. Preheat the oven to 375 F.
2. In a large mixing bowl, combine the eggs, almond flour, ricotta cheese, spinach, heavy cream, garlic, nutmeg, and paprika. Whisk together until well-combined.
3. Transfer the mixture to an oven-safe bowl.
4. Place the bowl in the oven and bake for 18 to 20 minutes, or until the mixture is no longer runny.

Keto-Friendly Overnight Oats

INGREDIENTS	Protein	Fat	Carbs
1 cup coconut milk	4.57 g	48.21 g	6.35 g
2 tbsp coconut oil	0 g	27.2 g	0 g
1/2 tbsp sunflower seeds	0.91 g	2.26 g	0.88 g
1 tbsp poppy seeds	1.58 g	3.66 g	2.48 g
1/2 tbsp chia seeds	1.32 g	2.46 g	3.37 g
1/2 tbsp almonds, slivered	1.69 g	3.99 g	1.72 g
1/4 tsp vanilla extract	0 g	0 g	0.14 g
3 tbsp protein powder	15.08 g	5.66 g	6.11 g

Nutrition Facts

Amount per 317 g
1 serving (11.2 oz)

Calories 976
From fat 792

	Amount	% Daily Value*	Amount	% Daily Value*
	Total Fat 93.4g	144%	Total Carbohydrates 21g	7%
	Saturated 68g	340%	Dietary Fiber 8g	33%
	Trans Fat 0.1g		Sugars 3g	
	Cholesterol 7mg	2%	Protein 25g	50%
	Sodium 142mg	6%		
	Calcium 41% • Iron 68%		Vitamin A 17% • Vitamin C 21%	

* Percent Daily Values are based on 2000 calorie diet. Your Daily Values may be higher or lower depending on your calorie needs.

INSTRUCTIONS:

1. In a blender, combine the coconut milk, coconut oil, and protein powder. Blend until smooth.
2. Transfer the contents of the blender to a jar with a removable lid.
3. To the jar, add the sunflower seeds, poppy seeds, chia seeds, and vanilla extract.
4. Mix until well-combined.

5. Cover the jar and refrigerate overnight.
6. Sprinkle slivered almonds over the oats before serving.

Ricotta Dumplings in Tomato Sauce

INGREDIENTS	Protein	Fat	Carbs
2 cups spinach	1.72 g	0.23 g	2.18 g
3/4 cup ricotta	20.94 g	24.14 g	5.65 g
1 egg	5.53 g	4.18 g	0.32 g
1/4 tsp nutmeg	0.04 g	0.22 g	0.3 g
1/2 cup peanut flour	15.66 g	0.17 g	10.41 g
1/2 cup tomato sauce	1.47 g	0.37 g	6.5 g
2 tbsp olive oil	0 g	27 g	0 g

Nutrition Facts

Amount per 470 g
1 serving (16.6 oz)

Calories 770
From fat 497

	Amount	% Daily Value*	Amount	% Daily Value*
Total Fat	56.3g	87%	Total Carbohydrates 25g	8%
Saturated	20.8g	104%	Dietary Fiber 8g	32%
Trans Fat	0g		Sugars 8g	
Cholesterol	259mg	86%	Protein 45g	91%
Sodium	901mg	38%		
Calcium 53% • Iron 28%			Vitamin A 145% • Vitamin C 43%	

* Percent Daily Values are based on 2000 calorie diet. Your Daily Values may be higher or lower depending on your calorie needs.

INSTRUCTIONS:
1. Bring a small pot of water to a boil over high heat.
2. Blanch the spinach on the boiling water for 1 minute. Remove the spinach from the water and set aside.
3. In a large mixing bowl, combine the spinach, ricotta, egg, nutmeg, and peanut flour. Mix together until well-combined.
4. Separate the dumpling mix into 5 equal portions. Form a small ball out of each portion.
5. In a frying pan, heat the olive oil over medium heat.

6. Fry the dumplings, making sure to turn them over occasionally to brown them on all sides. Cook each dumpling for 5 to 6 minutes.
7. To the same frying pan with all the dumplings, toss in the tomato sauce. Mix the sauce with the dumplings, making sure that they are all covered.
8. Transfer to a plate and serve immediately.

Roasted Vegetables in Pesto

INGREDIENTS	Protein	Fat	Carbs
1 small zucchini, cubes	1.43 g	0.38 g	3.67 g
5 spears asparagus	0.39 g	0.02 g	0.68 g
1/2 cup firm tofu, cubes	19.88 g	10.99 g	5.38 g
1/4 cup brussels sprouts, quartered	0.74 g	0.07 g	1.97 g
2 tbsp olive oil	0 g	27 g	0 g
2 tbsp pesto sauce	3.13 g	17.6 g	1.28 g
1/4 cup almonds, slivered	5.71 g	13.48 g	5.82 g

Nutrition Facts

Amount per 368 g
1 serving (13 oz)

Calories 782
From fat 601

	Amount	% Daily Value*	Amount	% Daily Value*
Total Fat	69.5g	107%	Total Carbohydrates 19g	6%
Saturated	9.4g	47%	Dietary Fiber 9g	36%
Trans Fat	0g		Sugars 5g	
Cholesterol	5mg	2%	Protein 31g	63%
Sodium	322mg	13%		
Calcium 104% • Iron 35%			Vitamin A 22% • Vitamin C 71%	

* Percent Daily Values are based on 2000 calorie diet. Your Daily Values may be higher or lower depending on your calorie needs.

INSTRUCTIONS:

1. Preheat the oven to 400 F.
2. On a baking tray, toss together the zucchini, asparagus, tofu, and brussels sprouts with olive oil. Season with salt and pepper if desired.
3. Bake in the oven for 20 to 25 minutes.
4. Remove the tray from the oven and transfer to a serving dish.
5. Drizzle with pesto sauce and sprinkle with slivered almonds before serving.

Keto Vegetarian Club Salad

INGREDIENTS	Protein	Fat	Carbs
3 cups romaine lettuce, shredded	1.73 g	0.42 g	4.64 g
1 egg	5.53 g	4.18 g	0.32 g
1 tomato	1.08 g	0.25 g	4.78 g
1 cup cucumber, cubes	0.78 g	0.21 g	2.87 g
1/2 cup cheddar, shredded	13.58 g	19.11 g	0.75 g
1 tbsp white onion, chopped	0.11 g	0.01 g	0.93 g
2 tbsp mayonnaise	0.26 g	20.66 g	0.16 g
1 tbsp olive oil	0 g	13.5 g	0 g
1 tbsp mustard	0.58 g	0.52 g	0.91 g
1 tbsp sour cream	0.42 g	1.27 g	0.85 g

<table>
<tr><td rowspan="2">Nutrition Facts

Amount per 576 g
1 serving (20.3 oz)

Calories 691
From fat 538</td><td>Amount</td><td>% Daily Value*</td><td>Amount</td><td>% Daily Value*</td></tr>
<tr><td colspan="4">
<table>
<tr><td>Total Fat 60.1g</td><td>93%</td><td>Total Carbohydrates 16g</td><td>5%</td></tr>
<tr><td>Saturated 18.3g</td><td>92%</td><td>Dietary Fiber 6g</td><td>25%</td></tr>
<tr><td>Trans Fat 0.7g</td><td></td><td>Sugars 8g</td><td></td></tr>
<tr><td>Cholesterol 237mg</td><td>79%</td><td>Protein 24g</td><td>48%</td></tr>
<tr><td>Sodium 805mg</td><td>34%</td><td></td><td></td></tr>
<tr><td>Calcium 52% • Iron 18%</td><td></td><td>Vitamin A 286% • Vitamin C 46%</td><td></td></tr>
</table>
* Percent Daily Values are based on 2000 calorie diet. Your Daily Values may be higher or lower depending on your calorie needs.
</td></tr>
</table>

INSTRUCTIONS:

1. Slice the egg into cubes or strips.
2. In a large bowl, combine the lettuce, cucumber, tomato, egg, white onion, and cheddar.
3. In a separate bowl, whisk together the mayonnaise, olive oil, mustard, and sour cream until well-combined.
4. Pour the dressing over the salad. Toss well.
5. Serve immediately.

Asparagus and Tofu Mash

INGREDIENTS	Protein	Fat	Carbs
6 spears asparagus	2.11 g	0.12 g	3.72 g
3/4 cup silky tofu, cubes	12.18 g	6.86 g	3.35 g
1 cup coconut milk	4.57 g	48.21 g	6.35 g
2 tbsp coconut oil	0 g	27.2 g	0 g
1 tbsp green onion, chopped	0.06 g	0.03 g	0.34 g
1 tbsp lemon juice	0.05 g	0.04 g	1.06 g
1/2 tbsp parsley, chopped	0.06 g	0.02 g	0.12 g

<table>
<tr><td rowspan="6">Nutrition Facts

Amount per 558 g
1 serving (19.7 oz)

Calories 818
From fat 697</td><td colspan="2">Amount   % Daily Value*</td><td colspan="2">Amount   % Daily Value*</td></tr>
<tr><td>Total Fat 82.5g</td><td>127%</td><td>Total Carbohydrates 15g</td><td>5%</td></tr>
<tr><td>Saturated 67.3g</td><td>337%</td><td>Dietary Fiber 3g</td><td>10%</td></tr>
<tr><td>Trans Fat 0g</td><td></td><td>Sugars 4g</td><td></td></tr>
<tr><td>Cholesterol 0mg</td><td>0%</td><td>Protein 19g</td><td>38%</td></tr>
<tr><td>Sodium 48mg</td><td>2%</td><td></td><td></td></tr>
<tr><td colspan="3">Calcium 28% • Iron 65%</td><td colspan="2">Vitamin A 23% • Vitamin C 29%</td></tr>
<tr><td colspan="5">* Percent Daily Values are based on 2000 calorie diet. Your Daily Values may be higher or lower depending on your calorie needs.</td></tr>
</table>

INSTRUCTIONS:

1. Cut the asparagus into small segments, about quarter of an inch long each.
2. In a small pot, heat the coconut oil over strong heat.
3. Add the cut asparagus and green onions. Cook for 4 to 5 minutes.
4. Pour in the coconut milk and bring to a boil.
5. Add the cubes of silky tofu. Allow to simmer for 10 minutes.
6. Turn off the heat and add the lemon juice and parsley.
7. Transfer the contents of the pot into a blender or food processor.
8. Blend until you get a smooth mash.
9. Transfer the mash to a bowl and serve immediately.

Broccoli Cheese Fritters

INGREDIENTS	Protein	Fat	Carbs
1 cup broccoli, chopped	2.57 g	0.34 g	6.04 g
1 cup spinach	0.86 g	0.12 g	1.09 g
1 cup cheddar, shredded	27.17 g	38.22 g	1.5 g
2 eggs	11.05 g	8.37 g	0.63 g

2 tbsp sour cream	0.84 g	2.54 g	1.7 g
1 tbsp garlic, chopped	0.54 g	0.04 g	2.81 g
1 tbsp peanut flour	1.98 g	0.02 g	1.32 g
1 tbsp lemon juice	0.05 g	0.04 g	1.06 g

Nutrition Facts

Amount per 374 g
1 serving (13.2 oz)

Calories 684
From fat 447

Amount	% Daily Value*	Amount	% Daily Value*
Total Fat 49.7g	76%	**Total Carbohydrates** 16g	5%
Saturated 26.3g	131%	Dietary Fiber 4g	16%
Trans Fat 1.4g		Sugars 3g	
Cholesterol 451mg	150%	**Protein** 45g	90%
Sodium 935mg	39%		
Calcium 94% • **Iron** 19%		**Vitamin A** 101% • **Vitamin C** 164%	

* Percent Daily Values are based on 2000 calorie diet. Your Daily Values may be higher or lower depending on your calorie needs.

INSTRUCTIONS:

1. Preheat the oven to 400 F.
2. Cook the chopped broccoli in a steamer for 15 to 20 minutes, or until tender.
3. Place the cooked broccoli and spinach in a food processor. Pulse until you get a very fine texture.
4. In a large mixing bowl, combine the ground broccoli and spinach mixture, eggs, spinach, sour cream, garlic, and peanut flour. Mix all the ingredients until well-combined.
5. Prepare a baking tray by lining it with parchment paper. Pour the mixture into the tray and pat it until it's flat. The fritters should be about half an inch thick.
6. Bake the fritters in the oven for 25 to 28 minutes, or until the top has become firm and golden brown.
7. Remove the tray from the oven. Break the fritters apart into small pieces and serve while hot.

Creamy Broccoli and Leek Soup

INGREDIENTS	Protein	Fat	Carbs
1/2 cup broccoli, chopped	1.28 g	0.17 g	3.02 g
2 tbsp leeks (white part), chopped	0.17 g	0.03 g	1.57 g
1 tbsp garlic, chopped	0.54 g	0.04 g	2.81 g
2 tbsp butter	0.24 g	23.04 g	0.02 g
1/2 cup heavy cream	1.23 g	22.2 g	1.67 g
1/2 cup vegetable broth	0 g	0 g	1.5 g
1/4 tbsp sour cream	0.11 g	0.32 g	0.21 g
1 tbsp parsley, chopped	0.11 g	0.03 g	0.24 g
1 cup soft tofu, cubes	16.24 g	9.15 g	4.46 g

Nutrition Facts

Amount per 526 g
1 serving (18.5 oz)

Calories 608
From fat 479

	Amount	% Daily Value*	Amount	% Daily Value*
Total Fat 55g		85%	Total Carbohydrates 16g	5%
Saturated 30g		150%	Dietary Fiber 2g	9%
Trans Fat 0.9g			Sugars 6g	
Cholesterol 144mg		48%	Protein 20g	40%
Sodium 719mg		30%		
Calcium 37% • Iron 21%			Vitamin A 53% • Vitamin C 84%	

* Percent Daily Values are based on 2000 calorie diet. Your Daily Values may be higher or lower depending on your calorie needs.

INSTRUCTIONS:

1. In a large pot, melt the butter over medium heat.
2. Add garlic and leeks. Stir while cooking until tender, about 3 to 4 minutes.
3. Add the broccoli. Cook for an additional 3 to 4 minutes.
4. Pour in the heavy cream and vegetable broth. Allow to come to a boil.
5. Lower the heat to a simmer. Add the soft tofu. Simmer for 10 minutes.

6. Transfer the contents of the pot to a blender. Blend until smooth.
7. Pour the soup into a serving bowl.
8. Drizzle sour cream over the top of the bowl and garnish with parsley. Serve while hot.

Baked Eggs in Collard Greens and Tomatoes

INGREDIENTS	Protein	Fat	Carbs
2 eggs	11.05 g	8.37 g	0.63 g
3 cups collard greens, chopped	3.26 g	0.66 g	5.85 g
2 tomatoes, diced	2.16 g	0.49 g	9.57 g
2 cups basil, chopped	1.51 g	0.31 g	1.27 g
1 tbsp olive oil	0 g	13.5 g	0 g
1/2 cup cheddar, shredded	15.87 g	22.32 g	0.88g

Nutrition Facts

Amount per 570 g
1 serving (20.1 oz)

Calories 603
From fat 408

	Amount	% Daily Value*	Amount	% Daily Value*
Total Fat	45.7g	70%	Total Carbohydrates 18g	6%
Saturated	17.5g	88%	Dietary Fiber 8g	32%
Trans Fat	0.8g		Sugars 8g	
Cholesterol	395mg	132%	Protein 34g	68%
Sodium	583mg	24%		
Calcium	86%	Iron 25%	Vitamin A 223%	Vitamin C 134%

* Percent Daily Values are based on 2000 calorie diet. Your Daily Values may be higher or lower depending on your calorie needs.

INSTRUCTIONS:
1. Preheat the oven to 400 F.
2. In a mixing bowl, toss together the collard greens, tomatoes, and basil in olive oil. Season with salt and pepper if desired.

3. Transfer the vegetables to a baking tray. Arrange the vegetables such that there are two slots for the eggs near the middle of the pan.
4. Crack the eggs into the slots, making sure that the yolks are intact.
5. Place the tray in the oven and bake for 10 to 15 minutes.
6. Remove the tray from the oven and sprinkle the shredded cheddar on top
7. Return the tray to the oven and bake for 2 more minutes.
8. Remove the tray from the oven and transfer the contents to a serving plate. Serve while hot.

Creamy and Cheesy Cauliflower Rice

INGREDIENTS	Protein	Fat	Carbs
1 cup cauliflower, chopped	2.05 g	0.3 g	5.32 g
1/2 cup broccoli, chopped	1.28 g	0.17 g	3.02 g
1/2 tbsp garlic, chopped	0.27 g	0.02 g	1.42 g
1 tbsp basil, chopped	0.09 g	0.02 g	0.07 g
1 tsp oregano, ground	0.16 g	0.08 g	1.24 g
1 tbsp butter	0.12 g	11.52 g	0.01 g
1/2 cup ricotta cheese	13.96 g	16.1 g	3.77 g
1/2 cup cheddar, shredded	13.58 g	19.11 g	0.75 g
1/2 cup heavy cream	1.23 g	22.2 g	1.67 g

Nutrition Facts	Amount	% Daily Value*	Amount	% Daily Value*
Amount per 416 g 1 serving (14.7 oz)	**Total Fat** 69.5g	107%	**Total Carbohydrates** 17g	6%
	Saturated 42.5g	213%	Dietary Fiber 4g	17%
	Trans Fat 1.1g		Sugars 5g	
Calories 808 From fat 615	**Cholesterol** 234mg	78%	**Protein** 33g	66%
	Sodium 631mg	26%		
	Calcium 77% • **Iron** 12%		**Vitamin A** 56% • **Vitamin C** 157%	

* Percent Daily Values are based on 2000 calorie diet. Your Daily Values may be higher or lower depending on your calorie needs.

INSTRUCTIONS:

1. Cook the cauliflower and broccoli in a steamer until tender.
2. In a food processor, combine the cooked cauliflower and broccoli, garlic, oregano, and basil. Pulse until you get a very fine texture. Set aside.
3. In a large pot, melt the butter over low heat.
4. Add the heavy cream, ricotta, and cheddar. Stir continuously until the mixture starts to boil.
5. Add the cauliflower rice mix to the pot. Stir well until the cheese sauce has been well-incorporated.
6. Transfer to a dish and serve while hot.

Spinach-Stuffed Portobello Mushrooms

INGREDIENTS	Protein	Fat	Carbs
3 whole portobello mushrooms	5.32 g	0.88 g	9.75 g
2 cups spinach, chopped	1.72 g	0.23 g	2.18 g
1 cup ricotta cheese	27.92 g	32.19 g	7.54 g
2 tbsp butter	0.24 g	23.04 g	0.02 g
1/2 tbsp garlic, chopped	0.27 g	0.02 g	1.42 g
1 tbsp basil, chopped	0.09 g	0.02 g	0.07 g

<table>
<tr><td colspan="2">Nutrition Facts</td><td>Amount</td><td>% Daily Value*</td><td>Amount</td><td>% Daily Value*</td></tr>
</table>

Nutrition Facts	Amount	% Daily Value*	Amount	% Daily Value*
Amount per 595 g	**Total Fat** 56.4g — 87%		**Total Carbohydrates** 21g — 7%	
1 serving (21 oz)	Saturated 35.4g — 177%		Dietary Fiber 5g — 19%	
	Trans Fat 0.9g		Sugars 7g	
Calories 711	**Cholesterol** 188mg — 63%		**Protein** 36g — 71%	
From fat 495	**Sodium** 462mg — 19%			
	Calcium 60% • **Iron** 20%		**Vitamin A** 152% • **Vitamin C** 31%	

* Percent Daily Values are based on 2000 calorie diet. Your Daily Values may be higher or lower depending on your calorie needs.

INSTRUCTIONS:

1. Preheat the oven to 400 F.
2. Remove the stems of the portobello mushrooms and clean them thoroughly with water. Pat them dry.
3. In a small mixing bowl, combine the spinach, ricotta cheese, butter, and garlic. Whisk together until well-combined.
4. Lay down the mushrooms cap side down on a baking tray. Stuff each mushroom with the spinach mixture.
5. Bake in the oven for 20 to 25 minutes, or until the mushrooms have become tender.
6. Remove from the oven and transfer the mushrooms to a dish. Garnish with chopped basil before serving.

Mexican-Style Cauliflower Rice

INGREDIENTS	Protein	Fat	Carbs
1 cup cauliflower, chopped	2.05 g	0.3 g	5.32 g
1 cup firm tofu, cubes	39.77 g	21.97 g	10.76 g
1 tbsp red onion, chopped	0.11 g	0.01 g	0.93 g

Ingredient			
1/2 tbsp garlic, chopped	0.27 g	0.02 g	1.42 g
1/4 cup tomatoes, chopped	0.4 g	0.09 g	1.75 g
1/2 tbsp hot chili peppers, chopped	0.08 g	0.01 g	0.38 g
1/2 tbsp paprika	0.17 g	0.15 g	0.65 g
1/8 cup avocado, sliced	0.37 g	2.68 g	1.56 g
2 tbsp olive oil	0 g	27 g	0 g
2 tbsp butter	0.24 g	23.04 g	0.02 g

Nutrition Facts

Amount per 497 g
1 serving (17.5 oz)

Calories 887
From fat 652

Amount	% Daily Value*	Amount	% Daily Value*
Total Fat 75.3g	116%	**Total Carbohydrates** 23g	8%
Saturated 22.1g	110%	Dietary Fiber 10g	42%
Trans Fat 0.9g		Sugars 4g	
Cholesterol 61mg	20%	**Protein** 43g	87%
Sodium 256mg	11%		
Calcium 177% • **Iron** 44%		**Vitamin A** 43% • **Vitamin C** 120%	

* Percent Daily Values are based on 2000 calorie diet. Your Daily Values may be higher or lower depending on your calorie needs.

INSTRUCTIONS:

1. Cook the chopped cauliflower in a steamer for 10 minutes, or until tender.
2. Place the cooked cauliflower and the tofu in a food processor. Pulse until you get a very fine texture. Set aside.
3. In a large pot melt the butter with the olive oil over medium heat.
4. Add the garlic, red onion, tomatoes, and peppers. Cook for 2 to 3 minutes or until fragrant.
5. Add the cauliflower and tofu mixture. Cook while stirring for 8 to 10 minutes.
6. Sprinkle with paprika. Cook for an additional 2 to 3 minutes.

7. Transfer the cauliflower rice to a bowl. Serve with sliced avocadoes on the side.

Arugula and Feta Cheese Salad

INGREDIENTS	Protein	Fat	Carbs
1 cup feta cheese, crumbled	21.32 g	31.92 g	6.14 g
1 cup spinach	0.86 g	0.12 g	1.09 g
1 cup arugula	0.52 g	0.13 g	0.73 g
1/4 cup cherry tomatoes	0.33 g	0.07 g	1.45 g
2 tbsp olive oil	0 g	27 g	0 g
1 tbsp balsamic vinegar	0.08 g	0 g	2.72 g
1 tbsp walnuts, chopped	1.88 g	4.63 g	0.75 g
1/2 cup cucumber, sliced	0.35 g	0.1 g	1.29 g

Nutrition Facts

Amount per 348 g
1 serving (12.3 oz)

Calories 723
From fat 562

	Amount	% Daily Value*	Amount	% Daily Value*
Total Fat	64g	98%	Total Carbohydrates 14g	5%
Saturated	26.5g	132%	Dietary Fiber 2g	10%
Trans Fat	0g		Sugars 11g	
Cholesterol	134mg	45%	Protein 25g	51%
Sodium	1412mg	59%		
Calcium 82% • Iron 16%			Vitamin A 86% • Vitamin C 31%	

* Percent Daily Values are based on 2000 calorie diet. Your Daily Values may be higher or lower depending on your calorie needs.

INSTRUCTIONS:

1. Bring a small pot of water to a boil.

2. Blanch the spinach for 1 minute. Remove immediately
    and submerge in ice cold water. Drain and dry
    thoroughly.
3. In a serving bowl, combine the blanched spinach, arugula,
    feta cheese, cucumber, and cherry tomatoes.
4. Drizzle the olive oil and balsamic vinegar. Toss the salad.
5. Sprinkle with chopped walnuts. Serve.
6.

Ricotta-Stuffed Bell Peppers

INGREDIENTS	Protein	Fat	Carbs
2 medium bell peppers	2.05 g	0.4 g	11.04 g
1 egg	5.53 g	4.18 g	0.32 g
1 cup ricotta cheese	27.92 g	32.19 g	7.54 g
1/2 tbsp garlic, chopped	0.27 g	0.02 g	1.42 g
1tsp oregano	0.09 g	0.04 g	0.69 g
1/2 tbsp chives, chopped	0.05 g	0.01 g	0.07 g
2 tbsp olive oil	0 g	27 g	0 g

Nutrition Facts

Amount per 564 g
1 serving (19.9 oz)

Calories 790
From fat 563

	Amount	% Daily Value*	Amount	% Daily Value*
Total Fat 63.9g		98%	Total Carbohydrates 21g	7%
Saturated 25.8g		129%	Dietary Fiber 5g	18%
Trans Fat 0g			Sugars 7g	
Cholesterol 290mg		97%	Protein 36g	72%
Sodium 280mg		12%		
Calcium 59% • Iron 17%			Vitamin A 46% • Vitamin C 323%	

* Percent Daily Values are based on 2000 calorie diet. Your Daily Values may be higher or lower depending on your calorie needs.

INSTRUCTIONS:
1. Preheat the oven to 350 F.
2. Slice the bell pepper in half and discard the seeds.

3. In a small mixing bowl, combine the egg, ricotta cheese, garlic, and oregano. Mix well until well-combined.
4. Lay the bell peppers down on the baking tray with their empty cavities facing up.
5. Stuff the bell peppers with the ricotta mixture, making sure to fill up each bell pepper close to the brim.
6. Place the baking tray inside the oven and bake for 15 to 18 minutes, or until the filling has set.
7. Remove from the oven and transfer the stuffed bell peppers to a dish.
8. Garnish with chopped chives before serving.

Refreshing Green Smoothie

INGREDIENTS	Protein	Fat	Carbs
1 cup coconut milk	4.57 g	48.21 g	6.35 g
2 tbsp coconut oil	0 g	27.2 g	0 g
3 tbsp protein powder	15.08 g	5.66 g	6.11 g
1/2 cup lettuce, shredded	0.37 g	0.06 g	0.61 g
1/4 cup avocado, cubes	0.75 g	5.5 g	3.2 g
1/4 cup cucumber, sliced	0.18 g	0.05 g	0.64 g
1/2 tbsp ginger, sliced	0.05 g	0.02 g	0.53 g
1 tbsp lemon juice	0.05 g	0.04 g	1.06 g

Nutrition Facts	Amount	% Daily Value*	Amount	% Daily Value*
Amount per 399 g 1 serving (14.1 oz) **Calories** 888 From fat 736	**Total Fat** 86.7g	133%	**Total Carbohydrates** 19g	6%
	Saturated 67.6g	338%	Dietary Fiber 6g	22%
	Trans Fat 0g		Sugars 3g	
	Cholesterol 7mg	2%	**Protein** 21g	42%
	Sodium 143mg	6%		
	Calcium 23% • **Iron** 61%		**Vitamin A** 36% • **Vitamin C** 40%	

* Percent Daily Values are based on 2000 calorie diet. Your Daily Values may be higher or lower depending on your calorie needs.

INSTRUCTIONS:

1. Combine all ingredients in a blender. Add 4 to 5 ice cubes.
2. Blend until smooth.
3. Serve while still cold.

Keto Muffin Sandwich

INGREDIENTS	Protein	Fat	Carbs
1/2 cup almond flour	10.05 g	23.72 g	10.24 g
1/4 cup peanut flour	7.83 g	0.08 g	5.21 g
1/4 tsp baking soda	0 g	0 g	0 g
1/4 cup coconut milk	1.14 g	12.05 g	1.59 g
2 eggs	11.05 g	8.37 g	0.63 g
1/4 cup cheddar, shredded	7.93 g	11.16 g	0.44 g
1 tbsp olive oil	0 g	13.5 g	0 g

Nutrition Facts	Amount	% Daily Value*	Amount	% Daily Value*
Amount per 255 g 1 serving (9 oz) **Calories** 815 From fat 595	**Total Fat** 68.9g	106%	**Total Carbohydrates** 18g	6%
	Saturated 23.5g	118%	Dietary Fiber 8g	33%
	Trans Fat 0.4g		Sugars 4g	
	Cholesterol 361mg	120%	**Protein** 38g	76%
	Sodium 701mg	29%		
	Calcium 43% • **Iron** 31%		**Vitamin A** 16% • **Vitamin C** 1%	

* Percent Daily Values are based on 2000 calorie diet. Your Daily Values may be higher or lower depending on your calorie needs.

INSTRUCTIONS:

1. Heat the olive oil in a frying pan over medium heat.
2. Fry 1 egg sunny side up. Set aside.
3. In a mixing bowl, combine the almond flour, peanut flour, baking soda, coconut milk, and the remaining egg. Mix well until you form a smooth batter.
4. Pour the batter into ramekin or a microwave-safe bowl. You may separate the batter into two portions.
5. Microwave the batter on high for 90 seconds.
6. Turn over the bowls on a plate. Tap on the bottom and the sides to loosen the muffins.
7. Assemble the sandwich. Place the sunny side egg between the muffins and sprinkle with shredded cheddar. Serve while hot.

Pumpkin and Ricotta Cheese Pancakes

INGREDIENTS	Protein	Fat	Carbs
1 cup pumpkin, cubes	1.16 g	0.12 g	7.54 g
1 egg	5.53 g	4.18 g	0.32 g
2 tbsp peanut flour	3.92 g	0.04 g	2.6 g
2 tbsp butter	0.24 g	23.04 g	0.02 g
1/4 tsp vanilla extract	0 g	0 g	0.14 g
1/4 tsp cinnamon powder	0.03 g	0.01 g	0.56 g
2 tbsp coconut oil	0 g	27.2 g	0 g
1/2 cup ricotta cheese	13.96 g	16.1 g	3.77 g

Nutrition Facts	Amount	% Daily Value*	Amount	% Daily Value*
Amount per 349 g 1 serving (12.3 oz) **Calories** 776 From fat 618	**Total Fat** 70.7g	109%	**Total Carbohydrates** 15g	5%
	Saturated 49.8g	249%	Dietary Fiber 2g	8%
	Trans Fat 1g		Sugars 4g	
	Cholesterol 288mg	96%	**Protein** 25g	50%
	Sodium 364mg	15%		
	Calcium 33% • **Iron** 13%		**Vitamin A** 228% • **Vitamin C** 18%	

* Percent Daily Values are based on 2000 calorie diet. Your Daily Values may be higher or lower depending on your calorie needs.

INSTRUCTIONS:

1. Cook the pumpkin cubes in a steamer for 20 minutes, or until they are very tender.
2. Mash the cooked pumpkin using a ricer or a fork. Set aside.
3. In a large bowl, combine the mashed pumpkin, butter, egg, peanut flour, vanilla extract, cinnamon powder, and ricotta cheese. Whisk the ingredients together until you get a smooth batter.
4. Prepare the frying pan by brushing it with coconut oil. Place over low heat.
5. Cook the pancakes one by one by ladling the pancake batter into the frying pan. Turn over the pancakes when bubbles start forming on the surface, which should take about half a minute.
6. Repeat the process until all the batter has been consumed.
7. Serve the pancakes as fresh as possible.

Caprese-Style Omelet

INGREDIENTS	Protein	Fat	Carbs
2 eggs	11.05 g	8.37 g	0.63 g
1 cup cherry tomatoes, sliced	1.31 g	0.3 g	5.8 g

	Protein	Fat	Carbs
1 cup mozzarella, shredded	24.83 g	25.03 g	2.45 g
2 tbsp olive oil	0 g	27 g	0 g
1 tbsp basil, chopped	0.09 g	0.02 g	0.07 g

Nutrition Facts

Amount per 379 g
1 serving (13.4 oz)

Calories 728
From fat 537

	Amount	% Daily Value*	Amount	% Daily Value*
Total Fat 60.7g		93%	**Total Carbohydrates** 9g	3%
Saturated 21.3g		106%	Dietary Fiber 2g	7%
Trans Fat 0g			Sugars 5g	
Cholesterol 416mg		139%	**Protein** 37g	75%
Sodium 835mg		35%		
Calcium 64% • **Iron** 15%			**Vitamin A** 52% • **Vitamin C** 35%	

* Percent Daily Values are based on 2000 calorie diet. Your Daily Values may be higher or lower depending on your calorie needs.

INSTRUCTIONS:

1. Whisk the two eggs until airy.
2. Add the olive oil to a frying pan and place over medium heat.
3. Pour the eggs to the frying pan. Cook for about half a minute or until the bottom has started to set.
4. Toss in the rest of the ingredients to the top of the eggs. Try to spread the ingredients as evenly as possible.
5. Cook the omelet for 1 more minute.
6. Turn off the heat. Fold the omelet towards the center and transfer to a dish.
7. Serve immediately.

Zucchini and Walnut Salad

INGREDIENTS	Protein	Fat	Carbs
1 zucchini	0.3 g	0.04 g	0.34 g
2 cups arugula	1.03 g	0.26 g	1.46 g

1/4 cup walnuts, chopped	4.46 g	19.11 g	4.02 g
1 tbsp sunflower seeds	1.83 g	4.53 g	1.76 g
2 tbsp olive oil	0 g	27 g	0 g
2 tbsp lemon juice	0.11 g	0.07 g	2.1g
1 tbsp mayonnaise	0.89 g	4.77 g	0.46 g
1/2 cup feta cheese, crumbled	10.66 g	15.96 g	3.07 g

Nutrition Facts

Amount per 237 g
1 serving (8.3 oz)

Calories 747
From fat 623

Amount	% Daily Value*	Amount	% Daily Value*
Total Fat 71.7g	110%	**Total Carbohydrates** 13g	4%
Saturated 17.6g	88%	Dietary Fiber 4g	15%
Trans Fat 0g		Sugars 6g	
Cholesterol 67mg	22%	**Protein** 19g	39%
Sodium 817mg	34%		
Calcium 48% • **Iron** 15%		**Vitamin A** 27% • **Vitamin C** 37%	

* Percent Daily Values are based on 2000 calorie diet. Your Daily Values may be higher or lower depending on your calorie needs.

INSTRUCTIONS:
1. Slice the zucchini into thin strips using a mandolin slicer.
2. In a large bowl, combine the sliced zucchini, arugula, walnuts, sunflower seeds, and feta cheese.
3. Whisk together the olive oil, lemon juice, and mayonnaise in a separate bowl until all components are well-combined.
4. Drizzle the dressing over the salad.
5. Toss the salad and serve immediately.

Quick and Easy Keto Yogurt Bowl

INGREDIENTS	Protein	Fat	Carbs
3/4 cup Greek yogurt	18.85 g	0.72 g	6.66 g

1/2 cup coconut milk	2.28 g	24.1 g	3.18 g
3 tbsp protein powder	15.08 g	5.66 g	6.11 g
1/2 tbsp sunflower seeds	0.91 g	2.26 g	0.88 g
1/4 tbsp chia seeds	0.66 g	1.23 g	1.68 g
1 tbsp almond butter	3.35 g	8.88 g	3.01 g
1/2 tbsp almonds, slivered	1.69 g	3.99 g	1.72 g

Nutrition Facts

Amount per 363 g
1 serving (12.8 oz)

Calories 657
From fat 396

	Amount	% Daily Value*		Amount	% Daily Value*
Total Fat 46.9g		72%	**Total Carbohydrates** 23g		8%
Saturated 23.4g		117%	Dietary Fiber 7g		27%
Trans Fat 0g			Sugars 9g		
Cholesterol 16mg		5%	**Protein** 43g		86%
Sodium 192mg		8%			
Calcium 50% • **Iron** 45%			**Vitamin A** 17% • **Vitamin C** 19%		

* Percent Daily Values are based on 2000 calorie diet. Your Daily Values may be higher or lower depending on your calorie needs.

INSTRUCTIONS:

1. In a blender, combine the Greek yogurt, coconut milk, almond butter, and protein powder. Blend until smooth.
2. Transfer the contents of the blender to a small bowl.
3. To the bowl, add the sunflower seeds, chia seeds, and slivered almonds.
4. Refrigerate the yogurt bowl for 1 to 2 hours to allow the chia seeds to swell.
5. Serve the yogurt bowl chilled.

Baked Ricotta Tarts

INGREDIENTS	Protein	Fat	Carbs
2 eggs	11.05 g	8.37 g	0.63 g
1/2 cup ricotta cheese	13.96 g	16.1 g	3.77 g

1/4 cup heavy cream	0.62 g	11.1 g	0.84 g
1 tbsp butter	0.12 g	11.52 g	0.01 g
1/4 cup peanut flour	7.83 g	0.08 g	5.21 g
1/4 cup cherry tomatoes, sliced	0.33 g	0.07 g	1.45 g
1 tbsp olives, sliced	0.07 g	0.9 g	0.53 g
1/4 tbsp garlic, chopped	0.13 g	0.01 g	0.69 g
1 tbsp chives, chopped	0.1 g	0.02 g	0.13 g

Nutrition Facts

Amount per 322 g
1 serving (11.4 oz)

Calories 616
From fat 425

Amount	% Daily Value*	Amount	% Daily Value*
Total Fat 48.2g	74%	Total Carbohydrates 13g	4%
Saturated 27.4g	137%	Dietary Fiber 3g	13%
Trans Fat 0.5g		Sugars 4g	
Cholesterol 462mg	154%	Protein 34g	68%
Sodium 423mg	18%		
Calcium 37% • Iron 16%		Vitamin A 46% • Vitamin C 13%	

* Percent Daily Values are based on 2000 calorie diet. Your Daily Values may be higher or lower depending on your calorie needs.

INSTRUCTIONS:

1. Preheat the oven to 400 F.
2. In a large mixing bowl, combine the eggs, ricotta cheese, heavy cream, peanut flour, cherry tomatoes, olives, and garlic. Mix until well-combined.
3. Prepare a muffin tray by brushing its surface with melted butter.
4. Pour the batter into the muffin tray. Make sure that each mold is filled close to the brim.
5. Bake in the oven for 15 to 20 minutes, or until the top of each muffin has set.
6. Remove the tray from the oven and transfer that ricotta tarts to a serving dish.
7. Garnish with chopped chives before serving.

Hearty Vegetable Soup

INGREDIENTS	Protein	Fat	Carbs
1/2 cup heavy cream	1.23 g	1.23 g	1.67 g
1/2 cup vegetable broth	0 g	0 g	1.5 g
1 tbsp butter	0.12 g	11.52 g	0.01 g
1 tbsp white onions	0.11 g	0.01 g	0.93 g
1/4 tbsp garlic	0.13 g	0.01 g	0.69 g
1/4 tbsp ginger	0.03 g	0.01 g	0.27 g
1/2 tbsp tomatoes	0.27 g	0.06 g	1.21 g
1/4 cup cauliflower, chopped	0.51 g	0.08 g	1.33 g
1/4 cup green beans, chopped	0.46 g	9.06 g	1.74 g
1/2 tbsp thyme	0.07 g	0.02 g	0.29 g
1/4 tbsp paprika	0.24 g	0.22 g	0.92 g
1/2 cup firm tofu, cubes	19.88 g	10.99 g	5.38 g

Nutrition Facts

Amount per 417 g
1 serving (14.7 oz)

Calories 532
From fat 392

Amount	% Daily Value*	Amount	% Daily Value*
Total Fat 45.2g	69%	Total Carbohydrates 16g	5%
Saturated 22.8g	114%	Dietary Fiber 6g	22%
Trans Fat 0.5g		Sugars 5g	
Cholesterol 113mg	38%	Protein 23g	46%
Sodium 615mg	26%		
Calcium 94% • Iron 25%		Vitamin A 60% • Vitamin C 40%	

* Percent Daily Values are based on 2000 calorie diet. Your Daily Values may be higher or lower depending on your calorie needs.

INSTRUCTIONS:

1. In a large pot, melt the butter over medium heat.
2. Add the white onions, garlic, ginger, and tomatoes. Stir while cooking until fragrant, about 3 to 4 minutes.

3. Pour the heavy cream and vegetable broth and bring to a boil. Lower the heat to a simmer.
4. Add the tofu, cauliflower, and green beans. Simmer for 10 minutes.
5. Add the thyme and paprika. Stir and continue simmering for 2 more minutes.
6. Ladle the soup to a bowl and serve while hot.

Creamy Pumpkin Soup

INGREDIENTS	Protein	Fat	Carbs
3/4 cup coconut milk	3.42 g	36.15 g	4.76 g
1/2 cup vegetable broth	0 g	0 g	1.5 g
1 cup pumpkin, diced	1.16 g	0.12 g	7.54 g
1/2 tbsp garlic, chopped	0.27 g	0.02 g	1.42 g
1/2 tbsp ginger, chopped	0.05 g	0.02 g	0.53 g
2 tbsp butter	0.24 g	23.04 g	0.02 g
1/4 tsp nutmeg	0.04 g	0.22 g	0.3 g
1/2 tsp paprika	0.17 g	0.15 g	0.65 g
1/2 tbsp pumpkin seeds	1.1 g	1.81 g	0.54 g
1/2 cup mozzarella, shredded	17.91 g	0 g	1.98 g

Nutrition Facts	Amount	% Daily Value*	Amount	% Daily Value*
Amount per 501 g 1 serving (17.7 oz) **Calories** 690 From fat 525	**Total Fat** 61.5g	95%	**Total Carbohydrates** 19g	6%
	Saturated 47.2g	236%	Dietary Fiber 3g	10%
	Trans Fat 0.9g		Sugars 5g	
	Cholesterol 71mg	24%	**Protein** 24g	49%
	Sodium 1107mg	46%		
	Calcium 62% • **Iron** 41%		**Vitamin A** 234% • **Vitamin C** 23%	

* Percent Daily Values are based on 2000 calorie diet. Your Daily Values may be higher or lower depending on your calorie needs.

INSTRUCTIONS:

1. Cook the pumpkin in a steamer for 15 to 20 minutes, or until it becomes very tender.
2. In a food processor, combine the cooked pumpkin, garlic, and ginger. Pulse until very smooth.
3. Melt the butter in a large pot over medium heat.
4. Add the coconut milk and vegetable broth. Stir and bring to a boil.
5. Add the pumpkin puree. Lower the heat to a simmer. Continue stirring while simmering for an additional 6 to 7 minutes.
6. Add the nutmeg and paprika. Stir and continue simmering for 2 more minutes.
7. Ladle the soup to a bowl. Top with pumpkin seeds and mozzarella. Serve.

Roasted Vegetables Smothered in

Pesto and Ricotta

INGREDIENTS	Protein	Fat	Carbs
5 spears asparagus	1.76 g	0.1 g	3.1 g

1/2 cup cabbage, chopped	0.57 g	0.04 g	2.58 g
1/2 cup broccoli, chopped	1.28 g	0.17 g	3.02 g
2 tbsp olive oil	0 g	27 g	0 g
1/4 tbsp garlic, chopped	0.13 g	0.01 g	0.69 g
1 tbsp lemon juice	0.05 g	0.04 g	1.06 g
3 tbsp pesto sauce	4.69 g	26.4 g	1.92 g
1/2 cup ricotta cheese	13.96 g	16.1 g	3.77 g

Nutrition Facts

Amount per 383 g
1 serving (13.5 oz)

Calories 760
From fat 613

Amount	% Daily Value*	Amount	% Daily Value*
Total Fat 69.9g	107%	**Total Carbohydrates** 16g	5%
Saturated 18.5g	93%	Dietary Fiber 5g	18%
Trans Fat 0g		Sugars 5g	
Cholesterol 71mg	24%	**Protein** 22g	45%
Sodium 563mg	23%		
Calcium 43% • **Iron** 21%		**Vitamin A** 40% • **Vitamin C** 116%	

* Percent Daily Values are based on 2000 calorie diet. Your Daily Values may be higher or lower depending on your calorie needs.

INSTRUCTIONS:

1. Preheat the oven to 375 F.
2. In a baking tray, toss the cabbage, broccoli, and asparagus with olive oil and garlic. Spread the vegetables along the tray evenly.
3. Bake in the oven for 10 to 15 minutes, or until tender.
4. In a small mixing bowl, combine the lemon juice, pesto sauce, and ricotta cheese. Whisk together until well-blended.
5. Transfer the roasted vegetables to a serving dish. Pour the pesto and ricotta sauce over the vegetables. Serve while hot.

Keto-Friendly Three-Cheese Pizza

INGREDIENTS	Protein	Fat	Carbs
1 cup cauliflower, chopped	2.05 g	0.3 g	5.32 g
1 egg	5.53 g	4.18 g	0.32 g
1/2 cup peanut flour	15.66 g	0.17 g	10.41 g
2 tbsp olive oil	0 g	27 g	0 g
3 tbsp tomato sauce	0.55 g	0.14 g	2.44 g
1/4 cup mozzarella, shredded	8.97 g	0 g	0.99 g
1/4 cup cheddar, shredded	7.93 g	11.16 g	0.44 g
1/4 cup ricotta cheese	6.98 g	8.05 g	1.88 g

Nutrition Facts

Amount per 377 g
1 serving (13.3 oz)

Calories 719
From fat 453

	Amount	% Daily Value*	Amount	% Daily Value*
Total Fat	51g	78%	Total Carbohydrates 22g	7%
Saturated	16.8g	84%	Dietary Fiber 8g	32%
Trans Fat	0.4g		Sugars 7g	
Cholesterol	234mg	78%	Protein 48g	95%
Sodium	629mg	26%		
Calcium	72% • Iron 16%		Vitamin A 24% • Vitamin C 91%	

* Percent Daily Values are based on 2000 calorie diet. Your Daily Values may be higher or lower depending on your calorie needs.

INSTRUCTIONS:

1. Preheat the oven to 425 F.
2. Cook the chopped cauliflower in a steamer for 10 minutes.
3. Place the cooked cauliflower in a food processor. Pulse until you get a very fine texture.
4. Squeeze out excess moisture from the ground cauliflower by pressing it between clean kitchen towels. Repeat this process two more times.

5. In a mixing bowl, combine the cauliflower, egg, and peanut flour.
6. Prepare a baking tray by lining it with parchment paper.
7. Place the cauliflower dough in the baking tray and press flat. Shape the dough into a circle.
8. Place the tray in the oven and bake for 10 minutes.
9. Remove the tray from the oven.
10. Spread the tomato sauce over the pizza crust.
11. Sprinkle the mozzarella, cheddar, and ricotta over the pizza. Try to spread them as evenly as possible.
12. Drizzle olive oil over the top of the pizza.
13. Place the baking tray back in the oven and bake for an additional 7 to 8 minutes, or until the cheese has become bubbly.
14. Remove from the oven.
15. Allow to cool for 5 minutes before serving.

Eggplant Fritters in Tomato Sauce

INGREDIENTS	Protein	Fat	Carbs
2 eggs	11.05 g	8.37 g	0.63 g
1 cup eggplant, cubes	0.8 g	0.15 g	4.82 g
1/4 cup peanut flour	7.83 g	0.08 g	5.21 g
2 tbsp olive oil	0 g	27 g	0 g
1/2 cup ricotta	20.94 g	24.14 g	5.65 g
2 tbsp tomato sauce	0.37 g	0.09 g	1.62 g
1 cup spinach	0.86 g	0.12 g	1.09 g

Nutrition Facts	Amount	% Daily Value*	Amount	% Daily Value*
Amount per 459 g	**Total Fat** 60g	92%	**Total Carbohydrates** 19g	6%
1 serving (16.2 oz)	Saturated 22g	110%	Dietary Fiber 6g	24%
	Trans Fat 0g		Sugars 6g	
Calories 772	**Cholesterol** 422mg	141%	**Protein** 42g	84%
From fat 530	**Sodium** 337mg	14%		
	Calcium 50% • **Iron** 22%		**Vitamin A** 85% • **Vitamin C** 21%	

* Percent Daily Values are based on 2000 calorie diet. Your Daily Values may be higher or lower depending on your calorie needs.

INSTRUCTIONS:

1. In a food processor, combine the eggs, eggplant, spinach, peanut flour, and ricotta cheese. Pulse until all components are well-incorporated.
2. Divide the batter into 4 equal portions. Shape each portion into a ball.
3. Pour the olive oil into a frying pan and place over medium heat.
4. Fry each fritter, making sure to turn them over to cook them evenly. Cooking time for each fritter is 8 to 10 minutes.
5. Place the fritters in a serving dish and dollop tomato sauce over the top. Serve.

Keto-Friendly Spinach Quiche

INGREDIENTS	Protein	Fat	Carbs
1 1/2 cup spinach	1.29 g	0.18 g	1.63 g
1 egg	5.53 g	4.18 g	0.32 g
1/4 cup heavy cream	0.62 g	11.1 g	0.84 g
1/2 cup peanut flour	15.66 g	0.17 g	10.41 g
1/2 cup cheddar, shredded	13.58 g	19.11 g	0.75 g
1/4 tbsp garlic	0.13 g	0.01 g	0.69 g

INGREDIENTS	Protein	Fat	Carbs
1/2 tbsp chives	0.05 g	0.01 g	0.07 g
1 tbsp butter	0.12 g	11.52 g	0.01 g
1 tbsp olive oil	0 g	13.5 g	0 g

Nutrition Facts

Amount per 237 g

1 serving (8.4 oz)

Calories 729

From fat 531

	Amount	% Daily Value*	Amount	% Daily Value*
	Total Fat 59.8g	92%	Total Carbohydrates 15g	5%
	Saturated 28.4g	142%	Dietary Fiber 6g	23%
	Trans Fat 1.2g		Sugars 4g	
	Cholesterol 293mg	98%	Protein 37g	74%
	Sodium 619mg	26%		
	Calcium 52% • Iron 16%		Vitamin A 118% • Vitamin C 24%	

* Percent Daily Values are based on 2000 calorie diet. Your Daily Values may be higher or lower depending on your calorie needs.

INSTRUCTIONS:

1. Preheat the oven to 425 F.
2. In a food processor, combine the spinach, egg, heavy cream, cheddar, peanut flour, garlic, and butter. Pulse until the ingredients are well-combined.
3. Prepare a muffin pan by brushing each mold with olive oil.
4. Pour the batter into the muffin pan. Try to fill each mold near to the brim.
5. Sprinkle the chopped chives over the top of each quiche.
6. Bake in the oven for 15 to 20 minutes, or until the top surface has become firm.
7. Remove the tray from the oven and allow to cool for 10 minutes.
8. Remove each quiche from the muffin pan and place in a dish. Serve while

Five-Minute Broccoli Cheese Soup

INGREDIENTS	Protein	Fat	Carbs
1 cup vegetable broth	0 g	0 g	3.01 g
1/2 cup heavy cream	1.23 g	22.2 g	1.67 g

	15.87 g	22.32 g	0.88 g
1/2 cup cheddar cheese, grated	15.87 g	22.32 g	0.88 g
1/2 tbsp garlic, chopped	0.27 g	0.02 g	1.42 g
1 cup broccoli, chopped	2.57 g	0.34 g	6.04 g
2 tbsp butter	0.24 g	23.04 g	0.02 g

Nutrition Facts

Amount per 485 g
1 serving (17.1 oz)

Calories 728
From fat 602

Amount	% Daily Value*	Amount	% Daily Value*
Total Fat 67.9g	104%	**Total Carbohydrates** 13g	4%
Saturated 41.2g	206%	Dietary Fiber 3g	10%
Trans Fat 1.7g		Sugars 5g	
Cholesterol 211mg	70%	**Protein** 20g	40%
Sodium 1601mg	67%		
Calcium 54% • **Iron** 5%		**Vitamin A** 66% • **Vitamin C** 138%	

* Percent Daily Values are based on 2000 calorie diet. Your Daily Values may be higher or lower depending on your calorie needs.

INSTRUCTIONS:

1. In a large saucepan over medium heat, melt some butter.
2. Add the chopped garlic and fry lightly for 1 minute.
3. Add the vegetable broth and heavy cream. Allow to boil while continuously stirring.
4. Add the chopped broccoli and grated cheddar. Cook for an additional 3 to 4 minutes or until the broccoli has turned bright green.
5. Serve while hot.

Traditional-Style Mediterranean Salad

INGREDIENTS	Protein	Fat	Carbs
1/2 cup cherry tomatoes	0.66 g	0.15 g	2.9 g

	0.35 g	0.1 g	1.29 g
1/2 cup cucumber, sliced	0.35 g	0.1 g	1.29 g
1 tbsp olives, sliced	0.07 g	0.9 g	0.53 g
1/4 cup red onions, sliced	0.32 g	0.03 g	2.69 g
1/2 tbsp garlic, chopped	0.27 g	0.02 g	1.42 g
1 cup feta cheese, crumbled	21.32 g	31.92 g	6.14 g
2 tbsp olive oil	0 g	27 g	0 g
1 tbsp cider vinegar	0 g	0 g	0.14 g

Nutrition Facts

Amount per 367 g
1 serving (13 oz)

Calories 686
From fat 529

Amount	% Daily Value*	Amount	% Daily Value*
Total Fat 60.1g	92%	**Total Carbohydrates** 15g	5%
Saturated 26.3g	132%	Dietary Fiber 2g	9%
Trans Fat 0g		Sugars 10g	
Cholesterol 134mg	45%	**Protein** 23g	46%
Sodium 1445mg	60%		
Calcium 78% • **Iron** 11%		**Vitamin A** 27% • **Vitamin C** 26%	

* Percent Daily Values are based on 2000 calorie diet. Your Daily Values may be higher or lower depending on your calorie needs.

INSTRUCTIONS:

1. In a large bowl, combine the cherry tomatoes, cucumber, red onions, olives, and garlic.
2. Whisk together the olive oil and cider vinegar in a separate bowl.
3. Drizzle the dressing over the salad.
4. Sprinkle the crumbled feta over the salad.
5. Toss well and serve.

Cucumber and Dill Salad

INGREDIENTS	Protein	Fat	Carbs
1 cup cucumber, sliced	0.7 g	0.19 g	2.57 g

	Protein	Fat	Carbs
1/4 cup red onion, sliced	0.32 g	0.03 g	2.69 g
1 tbsp dill weed	1.11 g	0.36 g	2.25 g
1/4 tbsp sour cream	2.01 g	6.1 g	4.08 g
1/2 cup ricotta cheese	13.85 g	15.97 g	3.74 g
2 tbsp olive oil	0 g	27 g	0 g

Nutrition Facts

Amount per 387 g
1 serving (13.7 oz)

Calories 570
From fat 439

	Amount	% Daily Value*		Amount	% Daily Value*
Total Fat	49.6g	76%	Total Carbohydrates	15g	5%
Saturated	17.8g	89%	Dietary Fiber	2g	8%
Trans Fat	0g		Sugars	3g	
Cholesterol	83mg	28%	Protein	18g	36%
Sodium	175mg	7%			
Calcium 43% • Iron 17%			Vitamin A 66% • Vitamin C 56%		

* Percent Daily Values are based on 2000 calorie diet. Your Daily Values may be higher or lower depending on your calorie needs.

INSTRUCTIONS:

1. In a large bowl, combine the sliced cucumber and red onion. Toss together.
2. In a separate and smaller bowl, whisk together the sour cream, ricotta cheese, and olive oil.
3. Combine the sour cream dressing with the salad. Sprinkle the dill weed over thc salad.
4. Toss well and serve.

Roasted Herbed Tofu and Mushrooms

INGREDIENTS	Protein	Fat	Carbs
1 cup portabella mushrooms, sliced	1.81 g	0.3 g	3.33 g
1 cup firm tofu, diced	39.77 g	21.97 g	10.76 g
2 tbsp olive oil	0 g	27 g	0 g

2 tbsp balsamic vinegar	0.16 g	0 g	5.45 g
1/4 tbsp garlic	0.13 g	0.01 g	0.69 g
1 tsp thyme, chopped	0.04 g	0.01 g	0.2 g
1 tsp parsley, chopped	0.04 g	0.01 g	0.08 g

Nutrition Facts

Amount per 401 g
1 serving (14.2 oz)

Calories 656
From fat 425

Amount	% Daily Value*	Amount	% Daily Value*
Total Fat 49.3g	76%	**Total Carbohydrates** 21g	7%
Saturated 7g	35%	Dietary Fiber 7g	28%
Trans Fat 0g		Sugars 7g	
Cholesterol 0mg	0%	**Protein** 42g	84%
Sodium 52mg	2%		
Calcium 174% • **Iron** 42%		**Vitamin A** 11% • **Vitamin C** 7%	

* Percent Daily Values are based on 2000 calorie diet. Your Daily Values may be higher or lower depending on your calorie needs.

INSTRUCTIONS:

1. Preheat the oven to 400 F.
2. In a large mixing bowl, combine the mushroom, tofu, garlic, olive oil, and balsamic vinegar. Toss together.
3. Spread the tofu and mushrooms over a large baking tray as evenly as possible.
4. Place the baking tray in the oven and bake for 25 to 28 minutes, or until the tofu has turned golden brown.
5. Remove the baking tray from the oven and allow to cool for 5 minutes.
6. Sprinkle the chopped thyme and parsley over the roasted mushrooms and tofu. Toss together.
7. Transfer the contents of the tray to a plate and serve.
8.

Keto Waffles

INGREDIENTS	Protein	Fat	Carbs
6 tbsp peanut flour	7.61 g	4.93 g	7.04 g

	Protein	Fat	Carbs
2 scoops protein powder	25 g	6 g	11 g
2 eggs	11.05 g	8.37 g	0.63 g
2 tbsp coconut oil	0 g	27.2 g	0 g
1/4 tsp baking powder	0 g	0.01 g	0.61 g
1/4 cup whole fat milk	1.92 g	1.99 g	2.92 g

Nutrition Facts

Amount per 250 g
1 serving (8.8 oz)

Calories 693
From fat 423

	Amount	% Daily Value*	Amount	% Daily Value*
Total Fat 48.5g		75%	**Total Carbohydrates** 22g	7%
Saturated 28.6g		143%	Dietary Fiber 5g	18%
Trans Fat 0.1g			Sugars 5g	
Cholesterol 338mg		113%	**Protein** 46g	91%
Sodium 278mg		12%		
Calcium 80% • **Iron** 49%			**Vitamin A** 46% • **Vitamin C** 35%	

* Percent Daily Values are based on 2000 calorie diet. Your Daily Values may be higher or lower depending on your calorie needs.

INSTRUCTIONS:
1. Combine all ingredients in a blender. Add a pinch of salt.
2. Blend until you get a smooth batter.
3. Pour the batter into the waffle pan and cook according to instructions.
4. Repeat step 3 until all the batter has been used.
5. Serve with a pat of butter, if desired.

Crispy Cauliflower Bites with Cream Cheese Dip

INGREDIENTS	Protein	Fat	Carbs
2 cups cauliflower, chopped	4.11 g	0.6 g	10.64 g
1 egg	5.53 g	4.18 g	0.32 g
1 1/2 tbsp peanut flour	2.92 g	0.03 g	1.94 g

Ingredient			
1 tbsp sesame seeds	1.64 g	4.9 g	0.94 g
2 tbsp olive oil	0 g	27 g	0 g
1 tbsp sunflower seeds	1.83 g	4.53 g	1.76 g
1/4 cup cream cheese	3.44 g	19.86 g	2.36 g
1 tbsp butter	0.12 g	11.52 g	0.01 g

Nutrition Facts

Amount per 380 g
1 serving (13.4 oz)

Calories 775
From fat 636

	Amount	% Daily Value*	Amount	% Daily Value*
Total Fat	72.6g	112%	Total Carbohydrates 18g	6%
Saturated	25g	125%	Dietary Fiber 7g	27%
Trans Fat	0.5g		Sugars 7g	
Cholesterol	258mg	86%	Protein 20g	39%
Sodium	445mg	19%		
Calcium 15% • Iron 17%			Vitamin A 28% • Vitamin C 172%	

* Percent Daily Values are based on 2000 calorie diet. Your Daily Values may be higher or lower depending on your calorie needs.

INSTRUCTIONS:

1. Preheat the oven to 350 F.
2. Crack the egg into a small bowl and whisk until smooth.
3. On a separate bowl, combine the peanut flour, sesame seeds, and sunflower seeds. Mix well.
4. Dip each piece of the chopped cauliflower in the whisked egg and coat with the peanut flour mixture. Repeat this step for all cauliflower pieces.
5. Place the coated cauliflower pieces on a baking tray and drizzle with olive oil.
6. Bake in the oven for 24 to 26 minutes, or until the cauliflower has turned golden brown.
7. Remove the baking tray and set aside.
8. Place the butter in a ceramic or glass bowl and microwave for 20 seconds.
9. Add the cream cheese to the butter and whisk together.
10. Serve the crispy cauliflower bites with the cream cheese dip on the side.

Cheesy Keto Bagels

INGREDIENTS	Protein	Fat	Carbs
1 egg	5.53 g	4.18 g	0.32 g
1 cup peanut flour	31.32 g	0.33 g	20.82 g
3 tbsp cream cheese	2.58 g	14.89 g	1.77 g
1 1/2 cup mozzarella, shredded	53.73 g	0 g	5.93 g
2 tbsp olive oil	0 g	27. g	0 g

Nutrition Facts

Amount per 344 g
1 serving (12.1 oz)

Calories 886
From fat 410

Amount	% Daily Value*	Amount	% Daily Value*
Total Fat 46.4g	71%	Total Carbohydrates 29g	10%
Saturated 13.5g	68%	Dietary Fiber 13g	50%
Trans Fat 0g		Sugars 9g	
Cholesterol 242mg	81%	Protein 93g	186%
Sodium 1589mg	66%		
Calcium 178% • Iron 16%		Vitamin A 33% • Vitamin C 0%	

* Percent Daily Values are based on 2000 calorie diet. Your Daily Values may be higher or lower depending on your calorie needs.

INSTRUCTIONS:

1. Preheat the oven to 400 F.
2. Combine the peanut flour and egg in a large mixing bowl. Whisk together until you get a consistency similar to paste.
3. In a separate ceramic or glass bowl, combine the cream cheese and mozzarella. Place the bowl in a microwave and microwave for 1 to 2 minutes, or until all the mozzarella has melted.
4. Allow the cheese mixture to cool for about 5 minutes, or until it's just hot enough to touch. Add the cheese mixture to the dough.
5. Knead the flour until you get a homogenous mixture.
6. Prepare the baking tray by brushing it with some olive oil.

7. Separate the dough into 2 or 3 portions and shape them into bagels on the baking tray. Brush the top of each bagel with some more olive oil.
8. Bake in the oven for 16 to 18 minutes, or until the bagels have turned light brown.
9. Remove from the oven and serve while warm.

Cream of Zucchini Soup

INGREDIENTS	Protein	Fat	Carbs
1 medium-sized zucchini, sliced	0.3 g	0.04 g	0.34 g
1/2 tbsp garlic, chopped	0.27 g	0.02 g	1.42 g
1/2 tbsp red onion, chopped	0.06 g	0.01 g	0.47 g
1 cup chicken broth	51.87 g	16.61 g	1.85 g
1/2 cup heavy cream	1.23 g	22.2 g	1.67 g
1/2 cup feta cheese, crumbled	10.66 g	15.96 g	3.07 g
2 tbsp sour cream	0.84 g	2.54 g	1.7 g
1/4 tbsp basil leaves, chopped	0.02 g	0 g	0.02 g

Nutrition Facts

Amount per 385 g
1 serving (13.6 oz)

Calories 828
From fat 509

Amount	% Daily Value*	Amount	% Daily Value*
Total Fat 57.4g	88%	Total Carbohydrates 11g	4%
Saturated 31.2g	156%	Dietary Fiber 0g	1%
Trans Fat		Sugars 5g	
Cholesterol 260mg	87%	Protein 65g	130%
Sodium 1720mg	72%		
Calcium 48% • Iron 19%		Vitamin A 35% • Vitamin C 10%	

* Percent Daily Values are based on 2000 calorie diet. Your Daily Values may be higher or lower depending on your calorie needs.

INSTRUCTIONS:

1. In a large pot, combine the chicken broth, heavy cream, garlic, red onion, and zucchini slices.
2. Bring the pot to a boil. Continue cooking for 8 to 10 minutes, or until the zucchini has become tender.
3. Transfer the contents of the pot to a blender. Blend until smooth.
4. Pour the contents of the blender into a serving bowl.
5. Drizzle the soup with sour cream and top with the crumbled feta and chopped basil leaves.
6. Serve while hot.

Creamy Two-Mushroom Soup

INGREDIENTS	Protein	Fat	Carbs
1 cup portabella mushrooms, diced	1.81 g	0.3 g	3.33 g
1 cup white mushrooms, sliced	2.16 g	0.24 g	2.28 g
1 cup heavy cream	2.46 g	44.4 g	3.35 g
1/4 tbsp garlic	0.13 g	0.01 g	0.69 g
1 cup vegetable broth	0 g	0 g	3.01 g
1/2 tbsp parsley, chopped	0.06 g	0.02 g	0.12
1/4 cup mozzarella, shredded	8.97 g	0 g	0.99 g
2 tbsp butter	0.24 g	23.04 g	0.02 g

<table>
<tr><td rowspan="6">Nutrition Facts

Amount per 572 g
1 serving (20.2 oz)

Calories 707
From fat 597</td><td>Amount</td><td>% Daily Value*</td><td>Amount</td><td>% Daily Value*</td></tr>
<tr><td>Total Fat 68g</td><td>105%</td><td>Total Carbohydrates 14g</td><td>5%</td></tr>
<tr><td>Saturated 42.3g</td><td>212%</td><td>Dietary Fiber 2g</td><td>10%</td></tr>
<tr><td>Trans Fat 0.9g</td><td></td><td>Sugars 9g</td><td></td></tr>
<tr><td>Cholesterol 231mg</td><td>77%</td><td>Protein 16g</td><td>32%</td></tr>
<tr><td>Sodium 1391mg</td><td>58%</td><td></td><td></td></tr>
<tr><td></td><td>Calcium 37% • Iron 5%</td><td></td><td>Vitamin A 65% • Vitamin C 9%</td><td></td></tr>
</table>

* Percent Daily Values are based on 2000 calorie diet. Your Daily Values may be higher or lower depending on your calorie needs.

INSTRUCTIONS:

1. Melt the butter in a large pot over high heat.
2. Add the garlic and the two types of mushrooms. Cook while continuously stirring until the mushrooms are tender, about 10 to 12 minutes.
3. Add the vegetable broth and heavy cream and stir. Bring to a boil and cook for an additional 5 to 6 minutes to reduce the liquid.
4. Transfer the soup to a serving bowl. While the soup is still hot, top it with shredded mozzarella.
5. Sprinkle chopped parsley over the soup and serve.

Spinach Feta Quiche

INGREDIENTS	Protein	Fat	Carbs
3/4 cup peanut flour	23.49 g	0.25 g	15.62 g
1 cup spinach, chopped	0.86 g	0.12 g	1.09 g
1 egg	30.52 g	23.11 g	1.75 g
1 tbsp cream cheese	0.86 g	4.96 g	0.59 g
1 cup feta, crumbled	15.99 g	23.94 g	4.6 g
1/2 tbsp green onion, chopped	0.03 g	0.01 g	0.17 g

Nutrition Facts	Amount	% Daily Value*	Amount	% Daily Value*
Amount per 448 g 1 serving (15.8 oz) **Calories** 849 From fat 466	**Total Fat** 52.4g	81%	**Total Carbohydrates** 24g	8%
	Saturated 27.3g	136%	Dietary Fiber 8g	31%
	Trans Fat 0.1g		Sugars 10g	
	Cholesterol 1020mg	340%	**Protein** 72g	143%
	Sodium 1535mg	64%		
	Calcium 80% • **Iron** 38%		**Vitamin A** 98% • **Vitamin C** 15%	

* Percent Daily Values are based on 2000 calorie diet. Your Daily Values may be higher or lower depending on your calorie needs.

INSTRUCTIONS:

1. Preheat the oven to 400 F.
2. Crack the egg into a small bowl and whisk. Mix half of the beaten egg with the peanut flour.
3. Mix the peanut flour and whisked egg well. Transfer this mixture to a muffin pan or an oven-safe bowl. Pat down the crust until you get an even thickness.
4. Bake the crust in the oven for 10 minutes. Remove from the oven and set aside.
5. In a food processor, combine the chopped spinach, cream cheese, feta cheese, green onion, and the remaining egg. Pulse just until all ingredients have been well-combined.
6. Transfer the filling mix to the top of the prepared crust.
7. Using a spatula, spread the filling evenly over the crust. Make sure that the top of the quiche is levelled.
8. Bake in the oven for 12 to 15 minutes, or until the quiche has become firm.
9. Remove from the oven and allow to cool for 10 minutes before serving.

www.ingramcontent.com/pod-product-compliance
Lightning Source LLC
Chambersburg PA
CBHW031126250726
48655CB00002B/534